TABLE OF CONTE

CW00738635

FAILURE TO CONCEDE A LACK OF ROBUST JUSTIFICATION......... 1

THE BMJ WHOOPING-COUGH ATROCITY.............................. 6

THE LEGACY OF JONAS SALK: MOST FAMOUS OF ALL VACCINE-TRIALS PRE-COVID19................................. 11

VAXOPEDIA.ORG AND *THE CHAMPION* TRIAL....................................... 19

A BILL GATES PRODUCTION: HERD-IMMUNITY DEMONSTRATION. 28

THE FLU VACCINE.................... 34

ANIMAL VACCINES................. 41

JENNER'S TIPS......................... 48

MY PROPOSED EXPERIMENTAL-DESIGN.................................. 54

THE DIAGNOSTIC PARADIGM.. 58

POLIO.. 66

THE MEDIA AND MEASLES....... 76

DISEASE-FEATURING CULTURAL-DEVASTATION........................... 79

GERM THEORY......................... 84

FROG APOCALYPSE.................. 90

COVID19: THE FLOWERING OF A DELUSION............................... 111

EPILOGUE............................... 123

Failure To Concede a Lack of Robust Justification

'... all the statistics of small-pox mortality, whether of London; of England, Scotland, and Ireland; of the best vaccinated Continental States; of unvaccinated Leicester; or of the revaccinated Army and Navy, without any exception, prove the absolute inutility of Vaccination; and I feel confident that every unprejudiced person who will carefully read these few pages, and will verify such of my statements as seem to them most incredible, will be compelled to come to the same conclusion.'

— Alfred R Wallace

You can google 'Alfred Wallace' the biologist to confirm instantly who he is/was: a towering scientific figure (independent conceiver of the theory of natural selection (first person to officially record the theorem in writing), spearhead of the original anti-compulsory-vaccination movement). The Order of Merit was the greatest honour Alfred Russel Wallace ever received. This award has been described as "quite possibly, the most prestigious honour one can receive on planet Earth." It was awarded to him by King Edward VII in 1908 "in recognition of the great services which you have rendered to Science." There are only 24 living individuals in the order at any given time, not including honorary appointees, and new members are personally selected by the reigning monarch of Great Britain. Darwin in fact did not receive any medal specifically for his contributions to the theory of natural selection, whereas Wallace received five of them. Here is a website dedicated to Alfred's legacy: https://wallacefund.myspecies.info/ and there is an active Facebook page under his full name which this website is linked to.

I believe I have found *the most peer-reviewed* literature specifically covering the debating involved with the Royal Commission's investigation of vaccination efficacy. "Resistors logic: the anti-vaccination arguments of Alfred Russel Wallace and their role in the debates over compulsory vaccination in England, 1870–1907" was published in the peer-reviewed journals, *Studies in History and Philosophy of Biomedical and Biological   Sciences* (https://booksc.xyz/book/17264081/c20b4b   or https://www.sciencedirect.com/science/article/abs/pii/S13698 48607000386?via%3Dihub).

The British government had set up a Royal Commission to judge the debate of vaccination effectiveness after some 50 years of the product being sold to many people (including the military). Alfred argued that the vaccine is not effective, as is elaborately accounted in one of his books (the copy I retrieved online was riddled with typos), *Vaccination: A Delusion*, which he produced due to—as he saw it—'the ignorance and incompetence displayed by the Royal Commission'. Why the Royal Commission didn't demand a trial of 50 unvaccinated vs 50 vaccinated prisoners, or 500v500, I don't know. We didn't think that way back then— scientifically, that is ... *ethically*, we certainly thought that way.

After the Royal Commission—three decades later in 1904, three years before Great Britain dropped mandatory vaccination—a man who, according to Wikipedia, is credited with establishing the discipline of mathematical statistics and is known as one of the most famous and contributing statisticians in history, Karl Pearson, 'published a critique of the typhoid vaccine that made advocacy for vaccination, and its chief proponent Almroth Wright, seem old fashioned, paternalistic, and ultimately unscientific'. The authors added in citation:

> By 1904, when Karl Pearson's statistical analysis of Wright's results concluded that the statistical justification for the technique was poor and that its routine use should be suspended until trials had yielded

unassailable data, even the BMJ had come around to the view that Pearson had a point.

The Pearson article in reference here is well worth a read, not because it derides pro-vaccinators (it doesn't), but because it shows correlation strengths, etc. (Report On Certain Enteric Inoculation Statistics Provided By Lieutenant-Colonel R.J.S. Simpson, C.M.G., R.A.M.C. By Karl Pearson, F.R.S., Professor of Applied Mathematics, University College, London):
https://www.ncbi.nlm.nih.gov/pmc/articles/PMC2355479/pdf/brmedj08194-0039.pdf

If the germ theory of disease is as real as we think it is, we surely wouldn't have vaccinated thousands of military personnel operating in Africa and India and then found out that we weren't so sure it was doing any good at all: he—the bacteriologist and immunologist—would have vaccinated 20 prisoners and compared the rate of typhoid fever to 20 unvaccinated prisoners after spraying the typhoid bacteria in the air of the containment the 40 prisoners were in (or putting it in their food) ... instead, it seems that the man who developed the discipline of mathematical statistics had to point out that no one had a robust indication of Almroth Wright's new vaccine's efficacy, and the military was using it in Africa and India. For leading proponents of vaccination, this was the end of using statistical arguments as the primary resort to discover evidence for any benefit from vaccination.

The final excerpt from the Resistors Logic article reads:

Modern pro-vaccinationists have the advantage of having a more developed science of immunology, and laboratory models of immunity that are more rigorous and accessible. However, all scientific demonstrations rely on interpretive frameworks that are assailable in particular when the underlying theory is not intuitive to broad sectors of the population.

To me, an unassailable indication would be consistent, statistical indications in controlled trials that the vaccinated are less likely to die and/or less likely to endure a higher incidence of *disease* (not less of one technical diagnosis).

Next, in these two graphs ahead, is some data I have collated in the earlier days of my study into this debate (as I was forming an opinion) ... I think the data presented on the graphs makes for a surprise to many people at this stage (2020): Why can't we see the impact of vaccination here—*or, can you?* :

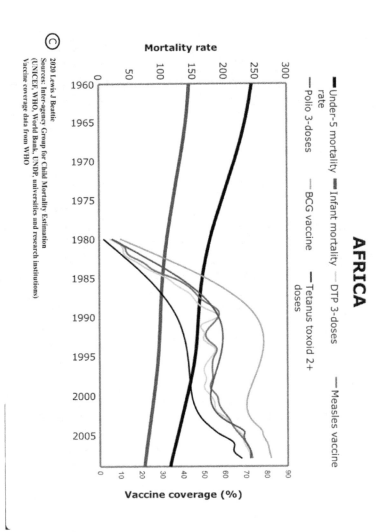

INDIA

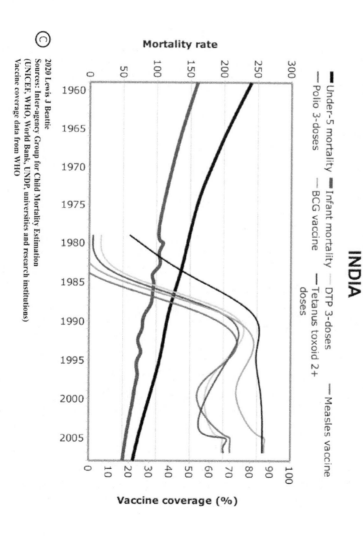

- Under-5 mortality ■ Infant mortality — DTP 3-doses — Measles vaccine
- Polio 3-doses — BCG vaccine — Tetanus toxoid 2+ doses

Sources: Inter-agency Group for Child Mortality Estimation
(UNICEF, WHO, World Bank, UNDP, universities and research institutions)
Vaccine coverage data from WHO

The BMJ
Whooping Cough Atrocity

A look at one of the earliest and biggest trials: a landmark trial. After many failed attempts by various different teams, this team appears claiming that success occurred, and the majority of the developed world agreed that that's what happened. I think the comparison of *vaccinated vs unvaccinated* was compromised in this specific trial. I'm calling it an *inadvertent abortion* because of *what was done to control for the placebo effect*. (Link to trial report: https://www.ncbi.nlm.nih.gov/pmc/articles/PMC2069253/pdf/brmedj03552-0003.pdf.)

Let's take a look at what the comparison group received (the "placebo"):

> The children in one group were inoculated with pertussis vaccine and are referred to subsequently as "vaccinated." Those in the other group were given a similar dose of "anticatarrhal" vaccine which contained no H. perttussis and are referred to subsequently as "unvaccinated."

> The "anticatarrhal" vaccine was prepared specially for the inquiry by Messrs. Burroughs Wellcome & Co. It contained killed suspensions of Staphylococcus aureus, Streptococcus pneumoniae, Corynebacterium hofmannii, and Neisseria catarrhalis, and was similar in turbidity to the plain pertussis vaccines.

Classical Gas
Soaking bacteria in formaldehyde/alcohol before injecting it inside your muscle might preserve its structure longer when it's in your muscle, and this would be good according to the vaccine theory. I'm reckoning that the micro-organisms in the vaccine had been soaked in formaldehyde (either before they were put into the vaccine and/or whilst in the vaccine) or some other form of preserving agent (as is often included in vaccines). The microbes from the placebo injection most likely weren't soaked in formaldehyde before being put/injected into the recipient, because *there's absolutely no reason for it*. For the microbes in the vaccine, we have an idealised reason for

it: We are supposedly *learning* from the microbes in the vaccine, and the longer they can preserve their essential genetic form in our body, the longer we can learn their essential genetic structure and develop defences against it, hence the placebo-injected microbes would have no reason to be soaked in formaldehyde—or something similar—at all. Formaldehyde would sap the microbial specimens of the majority of their festering/gas-producing ability before being inserted into the body; it forces the "juices" out of the micro-organisms.

The various species of dead bacteria that were injected into the placebo recipient were meant simply to shock the recipient's nervous system and consciousness so that they wouldn't know if they were vaccinated or not (imitating the effect of vaccination). Even if—*for some reason*—the microbes in the placebo injection *were* soaked in a preservative, or if the vaccine microbes and the placebo microbes weren't cured in a preservative alcohol-type solution, the placebo microbes may be more potent or more likely to rot inside the body in a way that makes the body more likely to develop a cough within this timeframe. The lungs are known as the second most excretory organ in the body:

> The lungs are part of the respiratory system [shown in the figure in the link below], but they are also important organs of excretion. They are responsible for the excretion of gaseous wastes from the body.
>
> https://flexbooks.ck12.org/cbook/ck-12-college-human-biology-flexbook-2.0/section/18.2/primary/lesson/organs-of-excretion-chumbio

Imagine ...
You have two dead baby mice, one that spent four weeks soaking in formaldehyde and the other freshly killed. The two mice would then be significantly different chemical packages. If you then insert the two differently-prepared mice into a

horse's muscle, they will probably decompose at a different rate, and in a different manner, thereby producing a different effect upon the chemistry and physiology of the horse. I daresay the mouse soaked in formaldehyde for four weeks would result in a less pronounced effect on the horse when injected into its muscle. There would be much more gaseous-build-up from the mouse that hadn't been soaking in formaldehyde.

Furthermore: Imagine that you have *a snail* and a mouse (quite different species, perhaps a similar chemical disparity to what was in the placebo and vaccine), and both weighed the same—do you think they would be likely to deteriorate and fester differently if we inserted them into a horse's muscle? Do you think they will produce a different effect upon the horse's physiological inclination to develop different genres of disease, as they are deteriorating inside? I do.

Do you think being injected with the placebo injection prepared by Messrs. Burroughs Wellcome & Co. makes for an appropriate representation of the unvaccinated body? I think saline solution, the kind people get IV-injected, would be an appropriate muscular injection for placebo-masking, and wouldn't cause *any significant gas* for one ...

Those who received this microbial cocktail injection were 4.5x more likely to develop a bad cough compared to those who received the vaccine. This was when whooping cough diagnoses were still made by clinical symptoms, not in accordance with a particular detection process, although that was just beginning to happen. Even if this vaccine did actually lower the recipient's chances of developing a cough—imagine this team did use a saline placebo injection and turned out these same results: *coughing aside*—did the vaccine increase their chances of *developing disease*, or *dying*?

This trial was part of the *ideological cementing process* after WWII.

We should have demanded stronger foundations before erecting such a huge ideological tower. In this BMJ medical report, this is what was said about the other so-called unsuccessful whooping cough vaccine trials:

> From 1942 to 1944 controlled trials were made in Oxford City with children attending welfare clinics and day nurseries, and also in Oxfordshire, Berkshire, and Buckinghamshire with children in residential nurseries. A report of this work was published by McFarlan, Topley, and Fisher (1945). No significant difference was observed in the incidence or severity of **the disease** between the vaccinated and unvaccinated groups. [Emphasis mine.]

The targeted microbe in this vaccine, accused of causing whooping cough at the time, has a different name nowadays. We used to think it was part of the Haemophilus family, but in the early 1900s they decided the differences were noticeable enough to give it a different family name, so we changed it to *Bordetella* after the guy who did most of the work therein, Jules Bordet.

I looked for the background rate of whooping cough surrounding this time, the closest to the age group and place of this trial that I could find: It looks like the notification rate was roughly equal to the rate found in the vaccine group, and the rate in the placebo-injected group was much higher.

Compare the kids in this trial (6–18 months old but followed for a couple of years, so we're looking at the 1–4-year-old age group) to the same group in the table on page three of the Eurosurveillance article shared a few sentences away. But remember, to get the rate, you take the rate per child a month and multiply it by 12 to get the rate per child a year.

Amirthalingam G, Gupta S, Campbell H. Pertussis immunisation and control in England and Wales, 1957 to 2012: a historical review. Euro Surveill. 2013;18(38):pii=20587. Available online:

For the BMC paper/trial under analysis here, I've calculated 1.45 x 12 = 17.4 in the vaccinated group, and 6.72 x 12 = 80.64 in the placebo. These rates were per 1000.

Contrast this with the Eurosurveillance data, which states that the notification rate in that age group during the last half of the 1940s was 22.4 per 1000. This is strikingly similar to the rate of the vaccinated group in the trial paper. But the placebo-injected group was roughly four times higher.

You may say, "Oh, but you can't compare two different data sets like that and claim an indication!" yet it still happens all over the world in 2020 and beyond, and it is *something*. Notification data is absolutely woeful. We don't know whether it under- or over-estimates the real occurrence of disease. Inclination, the initiative to report/notify surveillance centres fluctuates all the time; notification data is not data that is collected in order to assess vaccination efficacy.

The Legacy of Jonas Salk: Most Famous of All Vaccine Trials Pre-Covid19

Apparently, Jonas Salk was asked, "Why didn't you patent your vaccine?" to which he replied, "You can't patent the sun".

He seems to have been blackballed from the National Academy of Sciences, and there is debate as to precisely why though. Some say it's because at the initial press conference, after finally creating and trialling his vaccine, he never mentioned any of his team members' names. Some simply say it's because he was an unconventional scientist. I am convinced it's because his vaccine never provided any unassailable indication of its benefit. A trial was conducted and the vaccine appeared to be great—compared to a mystery-ingredients placebo injection—the media propagated this idea that the $5,000,000 trial (in the mid 1950s) was a great success before the American Statistical Association seemingly wrote the trial off as a huge waste of time and resources, and *not because the ingredients in the placebo were undisclosed*. This is perhaps why he was blackballed. His work didn't pass scientific scrutiny within the inner-circle scientific/mathematical community. It's easy to believe that no lies are told in this trial (as I personally believe), and the vaccine appears triumphant at first and second glance— although under rigorous scrutiny it seems there's no solid indication of benefit from this vaccine. This might be why his team was allegedly crying at the press conference, rather than the popular suggestion that their crying was due to him not mentioning their names (reference Sam Harris's *Making Sense* Podcast #158).

The big Salk trial
https://sci-hub.se/10.1001/jama.1955.02960140028004

Francis, T. (1955). EVALUATION OF THE 1954 POLIOMYELITIS VACCINE FIELD TRIAL. Journal of the

11

American   Medical   Association,   158(14),
1266.doi:10.1001/jama.1955.02960140028004

It's hard to find any trials conducted with the following: saline (placebo) injection vs vaccine; it's even harder to find trials including completely non-injected subjects compared to vaccinated subjects. The few I've found are included in this book—this trial is one of them. It included completely un-injected people, some mystery-ingredients placebo-injected people, and some polio-vaccinated people. A certain interpretation of the data from this very large-numbered trial speaks for the belief that the polio vaccine is one of the greatest human achievements. It went for one polio season, which is about three months. Inserted before this paragraph is a link in reference to the outcomes of the trial, but if that doesn't work you can find it somewhere in the world if you search for the heading of the trial which I've also included just before this paragraph started. A more detailed version of the study/report might be available in a library near you, although it appears to be rare.

This is what was said about what the placebo injection consisted of (I had to hunt down the full report of the trial, which resides in the library, to find this):

> A solution of similar appearance and composition except that it contained no inactivated virus or tissue products and should have no influence on immunity to poliomyelitis.

Note 'similar except' doesn't mean 'same except'. We are left to trust that the injection of these undisclosed ingredients in the placebo isn't at all conducive to the development of disease, not because the injection itself has been trialled in a large-numbered comparison to natural bodily terrain … in fact, it kind of has been now, with the further help after the trial of the American Statistical Association. Humans who were from a significantly lower socio-economic status were significantly less likely to develop paralytic disease than the humans who received the placebo injection … this is extremely suspicion-arousing of the placebo injection, begging the question "precisely what is it?" which seemingly nobody can answer anymore. From a time when the neurotoxic DDT was widely used (and even sprayed upon children, as many people know occurred, with some photographic accounts), we are left to trust that whatever these people used to simulate an immune shock was 100% all good. Someone has argued to me that the kids with lower socio-economic status are more resilient to polio because they encounter it earlier on in life, without referring to a specific study that found this occurs for the same-aged children in this trial (i.e. from what he is arguing, it could go either way). Either way, imagine if we ran the big COVID19 vaccine trials with mystery-ingredients placebo injections—it surely wouldn't happen nowadays.

The placebo-injected group had a significantly higher rate of paralytic disease than the un-injected, and were only-notably from a higher socio-economic status: this is what the AMA Professor Brownlee found when he scrutinised the trial, after the whole world was cheering-on Jonas Salk (the public was, the scientific community wasn't, and no one knows exactly why—some people even say it's because he was *a weird person*). There is a breach of statistical expectations here, and I think this is what Professor K.A Brownlee alluded to when he wrote in his report 'contains internal evidence of bias in favour of the vaccinated'. I've included a link to Brownlee's critique/article several paragraphs away, where I share my legal 10% of it.

The only mortality data reported was the fatal cases of polio. The placebo group consisted of over 201 thousand humans, with 162 cases of polio, and four fatal cases. The un-injected (and poorer) portion of the trial consisted of over 338 thousand humans, with 182 cases of polio, and no fatal cases. This, to me, indicates something is likely to be off with the placebo injection, and we should know precisely what was in it to get to the bottom of that. The Statistical Association only found a significant confounder in those un-injected being from a lower socio-economic status, which to me undermines the original Salk vaccine trial report, which had already been broadcasted across the world.

It isn't a conspiracy thing to suggest DDT was used as the placebo, it's just something that I feel would have been seemingly reasonable to those humans in the setting of 1954. We should be able to see the overall mortality rates of the polio-vaccinated and all the other children.

If we had access to the overall mortality rate, or a measure of overall disease-incidence, we could get a more accurate indication as to the dominant effect induced in this experiment: whether the placebo injection increased disease or the vaccine decreased it. Perhaps the placebo group's overall mortality rate (excluding polio deaths) was just as high or significantly higher than the vaccine group than it was for the polio rate. Perhaps Thomas Francis saw this and decided "It is a complex world, and here we are looking at *polio*". This is probably the strongest indication we could attain as to whether or not the placebo ingredients were actually poorly understood in their effect on health and disease (like DDT was at the time and many things are still now, I'd say).

Perhaps there is a drug or procedure that will lower the likelihood that people will develop a paralytic disease within three months. No drug has demonstrated this specifically as far as I know, although this major polio vaccine trial report seems to have claimed that's what happened ... you can analyse it, as the public did 70 years ago, with the added benefit of a report from the American Statistical Association— a benefit that came after the big media report of success— and you might agree with me that it doesn't *prove* anything of the sort. *If it did*, we should also want to be sure that we aren't trading one likelihood for another over at least one full year, to be reasonable. Paralytic disease is the window of focus for these three months. Just to reiterate: perhaps we can find a drug that will lower the chances of a certain genre of disease manifesting in 3–12 month; if there is such a drug, we should be keen to see if it doesn't increase overall disease incidence or mortality as we mitigate the one genre of disease.

For some reason, a lot of faults regarding the structure of this trial were realised only after it was conducted, after 5 million 1950's-US-dollars was spent, after the big media hype, during the thorough investigation conducted by the American Statistical Association (I've included a link and reference to this ahead).

Here is an excerpt from this polio trial report, from the medical association (the "uninoculated" are the completely un-injected; they were those whose parents declined the injection-participation):

> The question has been asked why the incidence of paralytic cases is less in the uninoculated members of the population than in the placebo controls. One can only repeat that the populations receiving vaccine or placebo are strictly comparable in every characteristic; they are equal parts of one population, while those who refused participation are distinctly different.

'Strictly comparable'—only we have no idea what the placebo recipients were injected with.

After this vaccine was mass-inseminated, doctors only diagnosed polio (which they surely had vaccinated most of their patients *against*) if the patient was paralysed, according to the guidelines they were advised to follow, including laboratory virus confirmation which was just becoming more accessible... quote: 'to avoid unwarranted criticism of the vaccine' (The Medical Journal of Australia *July 28, 1956 p158,* under the heading 'DIAGNOSTIC CRITERIA FOR POLIOMYELITIS').

Here is a link to the American Statistical Association's review of this trial *after* it was conducted and cheered-about ((K. A. Brownlee (1955) Statistics of the 1954 Polio Vaccine Trials*, Journal of the American Statistical Association, 50:272, 1005-

1013,   DOI:10.1080/01621459.1955.10501286
http://dx.doi.org/10.1080/01621459.1955.10501286).

As Professor Brownlee puts it:

> From the layman's point of view, probably the most interesting and convincing set of data is that which refers to the poliomyelitis cases categorized as paralytic and not-paralytic and not-polio. Since the paralytic cases are those for which there is the least difficulty in diagnosis we are probably justified in having greatest confidence in that part of the data, though some may prefer to consider only those cases confirmed by the laboratory.

The American Statistical Association seems to find the trial design and study to be myopic and resource wasting. It does suggest that some of the trial is *worth considering*. It was only because someone (uncredited) realised a blunder during the trial that they changed the settings, after disregarding one branch of the trial: 'only 41 per cent of the trial was rescued and the remaining 59 per cent blundered along its stupid and futile path'.

This paper is well worth the read; it's interesting to me the way this highly renowned statistician critiques the trial and initial report. I could copy and paste the whole thing here (if I had permission), but the paper is readily available online. The analysis goes on with many reasons why this is not a well-thought-out trial, which produces an outcry as to why this wasn't thought-out beforehand with the Statistical Association before spending five million dollars circa1954. Brownlee appears to be reprimanding the authors of the report for claiming to have found statistical significance where the professor of statistics found there was none, several times, and making all kinds of small miscalculations throughout the whole report, as is noted in the paper.

Here are some excerpts from the review:

> What for example, is one to make of [page 5]:

"In observed areas where only those second grade children whose parents requested participation were vaccinated, the problem of establishing the control population was more complex."

It is perfectly true to say that it is "more complex," but to indulge in understatements of this order of magnitude is to be misleading. The plain fact is that it is impossible. Why not say so? Continuing:

"After careful consideration of various alternatives, it was decided that the total first and third grade study population compared to the vaccinated second grade population would be the most critical measure that could be applied to measure the efficacy of the vaccine."

When the "most critical measure" is worthless, why allow the uninformed reader to continue with the impression that it is worth something?

The failure to face up to the implications of the confounding of vaccination status with age and other factors is manifested in the discussion of the data [page 27]:

"The unqualified attribution of these 'significance levels' to vaccination rather than to the complex of factors differentiating the two populations must be condemned."

"There is no need, in the pages of this Journal, to discuss the reasons for the need for randomization in experiments of this type, but it is perhaps worthy of note that this Report contains two very good illustrations of its necessity."

"The second place where the data of the Report make plain the need for strict randomization is in Table 2b, where, in the placebo area, those receiving the placebo had a significantly higher rate (57 per 100,000) of paralytic polio, than those not participating in the trial (36 per 100,000). A sample survey (page 13) established that the non-participants belonged to lower socio-economic groups than the participants."

"To summarize, 59 per cent of the trial was worthless because of the lack of adequate controls. The remaining 41 per cent may be all right but contains internal evidence of bias in favour of the vaccinated."

17

"The reviewer may seem too skeptical in feeling the need for an independent confirmation of a trial run on the scale of the present one, but **he would point out that gamma globulin was triumphantly proclaimed effective by the National Foundation after a similar trial, but now considerable doubts exist as to the correctness of this conclusion.**" (Bold emphasis mine)

VAXOPEDIA.ORG AND *THE CHAMPION* TRIAL

Quote: 'Have you ever heard that there are no double-blind, placebo-controlled randomised clinical trials for vaccines?

It isn't true.' end quote*:*
https://vaxopedia.org/2017/07/10/where-are-the-double-blind-placebo-controlled-randomized-trials-about-vaccines/

Here we shall analyse a trial championed by a prominent pro-vax website as the gold standard (this is seemingly *the* champion trial). The address above leads to the website and article in reference for this part of the book. Here is another quote from that exact location in the website address/link: "Tragically, many more folks got pneumonia and died if they got the saline placebo instead of the vaccine in this study."

Here is a link to the BMJ trial report of the "study" in reference of the *vaxopedia.org* article I am quoting:

https://www.bmj.com/content/340/bmj.c1004?fbclid=IwAR1DX ZFXqaQzFXz4X887YvnbSghUSgxZRmVO7m_SKsyYcS5u2 G_D-dddJuc

Nursing home residents were put through a well-controlled comparative trial to assess the effect of—what was considered the most important kind of—vaccination in nursing homes, for a bacteria called *pneumococcus pneumonia* which, according to reputable sources, (Janssens JP, Krause KH. Pneumonia in the very old. Lancet Infect Dis2004;4:112-24. Maruyama T, Niederman MS, Kobayashi T, Kobayashi H, Takagi T, D'Alessandro-Gabazza CN, et al. A prospective comparison of nursing home-acquired pneumonia with hospital-acquired pneumonia in non-intubated elderly. Respir Med2008;102:1287-95. Lim WS, Macfarlane JT. A prospective comparison of nursing home acquired pneumonia with community acquired pneumonia. Eur Respir J2001;18:362-8.) is the most critical and deadly microbe in the nursing-home setting—and the vaccination allegedly worked! If it did work, we should be primarily concerned if it worked for an overall better.

The ability to suppress or divert physiological functions (medicine, per se) dates back thousands of years. When people noticed that introducing metals to the body could alter the course of disease, this was one of the original microbial mitigation techniques, although the practitioners were not aware of the micro-organisms. Mercury and copper have been used in this way throughout history. Interesting story: apparently, the first emperor of unified China was prescribed some kind of mercury-based medicine in the hopes that it would prolong his life. Mercury application can probably hastens the speed in which superficial skin-cuts heal.

What we are analysing here is a vaccine trial from our day and age: it began in 2009, in Japan, as *an attempt to dispel vaccination infidelity*. When I first saw the headline, I wondered if I had finally stumbled upon what I was looking for (a trial that indicated that vaccination improved survival), as you might see why given what we have thus far seen from the BMJ trial report title and the *vaxpedia.org website's lofty tone* in presenting *the* champion trial... this is the BMJ report title:

Maruyama Takaya, Taguchi Osamu, Niederman Michael S, Morser John, Kobayashi Hiroyasu, Kobayashi Tetsu et al. Efficacy of 23-valent pneumococcal vaccine in preventing pneumonia and improving survival in nursing home residents: double blind, randomised and placebo controlled trial *BMJ* 2010; 340 :c1004

Because most vaccination trials use another vaccine as the placebo, this is apparently the champion trial for the crux of the debate; the website is basically saying, "Hey all you nae-sayers saying vaccination trials don't feature proper placebo controls, here's your saline placebo!". This is a brilliant trial because pro-vax people love it, and so do I, as the headline shows <u>how</u> this idea *vaccination saves lives* is claimed *as if it's an established fact.*

Saline seems to be the most chemically negligible compound we can inject inside the body at low doses, which provides enough of a shock to the recipient to work as a placebo mask.

So much for the common rebuttal that "we can't run such comparative trials, because too many unvaccinated people will die and it would be very unethical"—we have one here as the main display on a pro-vaccination website, and, for whatever reason, the vaccinated group had a higher death-rate. Furthermore, we have many animal vaccines which could show the lifesaving effect of vaccination in a controlled trial if it does exist, and yet when we decide to break this apparently-ethical code and run a controlled vaccination-trial to prove the overall benefit, we use *placebo-needing humans* rather than animals, and the vaccinated have a higher death rate …

Here are some more quotes from this vaxopedia.org article:

> So why haven't placebo control studies been done even more routinely then?
>
> Why isn't <u>every vaccine</u> on the immunization schedule or every combination of vaccines tested using a double-blind, saline placebo controlled study?"
>
> Placebo use in vaccine trials is clearly acceptable when (a) no efficacious and safe vaccine exists and (b) the vaccine under consideration is intended to benefit the population in which the vaccine is to be tested. Placebo use in vaccine trials: Recommendations of a WHO expert panel.
>
> Of course, the answer is that in order to do this type of study, you would have to have a very good justification for leaving many of the kids unprotected and at risk for a <u>vaccine-preventable disease</u>.
>
> Instead, as is discussed in the article "Current topics in research ethics in vaccine studies," if a vaccine is "already in use in some other country

or community which is more or less comparable to site where the trial is planned, that vaccine should be used as the comparator."

So, instead of a placebo, it is more common "to give another vaccine that provides comparable benefit against another disease, or more willingly, against similar disease caused by different agents."

When can you use a placebo control?

The article states that "placebo controls are ethically acceptable when there is no proven vaccine for the indication for which the candidate vaccine is to be tested." But get educated and don't be fooled, many double-blind, placebo-controlled randomized clinical trials have been done with vaccines."

https://vaxopedia.org/2017/07/10/where-are-the-double-blind-placebo-controlled-randomized-trials-about-vaccines/

This trial included 502 vaccinated patients and 504 *saline placebo injected* patients. Both groups were randomised so that they were equal in outcome expectations (the vaccinated versus the unvaccinated: a balanced composition of ages, weights, heights, health statuses, locations and perhaps even things like *ethnicities*). It is observed that the vaccinated humans in the trial were significantly less-likely to have died with a positive detection for the antigenic signature (urinary particle) of *pneumococcus pneumoniae*, fitting the criteria for a diagnosis of pneumococcus pneumonia: 14 received the diagnosis and 0 died, compared to the unvaccinated, of which 37 received the diagnosis and 13 died.

From the BMJ trial report: 'The participants in this study were at high risk of pneumococcal pneumonia. A sensitive and specific urinary antigen test was used to determine the efficacy of the vaccine.'

The vaccinated were more likely to die if they had this character of disease (pneumonia) *without* a positive detection-result for *P. pneumoniae*: 9.8% (49 out of 502) of the vaccinated people were diagnosed with non-pneumococcal pneumonia and 13.3% (67 out of 504) of the unvaccinated were diagnosed with non-pneumococcal pneumonia; of those who were diagnosed with non-pneumococcal pneumonia, 26.5% (13 out of 49) of the vaccinated died whilst 19.4% (13 out of 67) of the unvaccinated died.

Did it improve survival?
If we sample a random person's data from this trial—and they happened to have died—there is a higher chance that the dead person was one of the vaccinated. The only indication we have of *outright disease incidence* in this trial is in the mortality figures.

One idea that is backed up in the data from this trial is that when the respiratory cellular structures degenerated, the usual undertaking microbes were discouraged from undertaking these cells in the vaccinated, and this led to worse problems for the organism. Another idea I have is that the vaccinated body was more prone to degeneration/falling in general, but the biochemical *condition* the body was in after vaccination made for a different course of failing/degeneration/illness, leaving it less likely to produce urine that would have these specific particles detected in it (instead of pneumonia perhaps the respiratory cells developed cancer or maybe there was something else occurring in the body that took up all the physiological energy and diverted a pneumonic process).

Just as the world is not black and white, body chemistry / disease genesis is not simple—we probably shouldn't be thinking that because the vaccinated body was less likely to develop one specific character of disease *and/or a specific urinary particle* that it was better-off overall. The vaccinated body in this trial was clearly chemically-altered, for better or worse I don't know, we have no indication other than the mortality data, but it seems obvious-enough to me that mitigating one character of disease isn't an outright gain, as the intervention may have made a different character of disease more likely to erupt. How can we rule this out? We study all the disease symptoms …

The significance: It has been hypothesised that this vaccine reduces deaths—and we've found *evidence* that it does—from pneumococcal pneumonia for this disease, which is diagnosed with the criterion of *specific bacterial strain presence.* Although the death rate from non-pneumococcal pneumonia is higher in the vaccinated, the vaccinated group was seemingly spared 13 pneumococcal-pneumonia deaths due to the vaccine, as that's how many the saline group had, whilst the vaccinated had none.

If we accept that the vaccine does nothing other than lower the chances of pneumococcus pneumonia developing and killing the human, and look at the disparity in the mortality figures, this is found to be "statistically significant". Let's accept that the vaccine saved 13 lives (from pneumococcal pneumonia) and did nothing else. Take a look at overall deaths: the unvaccinated group had 80. So, using them as a benchmark, we theoretically expect to find 13 fewer deaths in the vaccinated group (80 - 13 = 67). Instead of 67 there were 89 deaths—that's a difference/discrepancy of 22 deaths between what we theoretically expect and what we've found. This difference is, by any statistician's definition, *statistically significant* (p=0.027, one-tailed).

Imagine if I told you that I could significantly lower your car's chances of *overheating* by putting a special engine-oil in it, and I showed you the experimental data where this was indicated … If the data I showed you included data showing how many cars broke down overall in any way (including overheating), and more cars broke down in the group that received the special engine oil, what would you think of that? Would you wonder if there's any way the special engine oil product could have contributed to the cars in the experiment breaking down in any way not related to overheating? Would you expect that these mechanics had run many large-numbered comparative experiments to clear up whether or not the special engine oil product increased the vehicle's chances of breaking down overall?

Excerpt from the BMJ trial report:

> We originally hypothesised that the vaccine would be effective only against pneumococcal pneumonia and not all cause pneumonia. However, even though all cause pneumonia and pneumococcal pneumonia were significantly more common in the placebo group than vaccine group, the death rates from all cause pneumonia and non-pneumococcal pneumonia and the incidence of non-pneumococcal pneumonia were not significantly reduced in the vaccine group.

Pneumococcal pneumonia is included in all cases of pneumonia. The incidence and death rate for pneumococcal pneumonia was significantly lower in the vaccinated. The death rate of all cause pneumonia wasn't significantly reduced in the vaccinated, even though this included death from pneumococcal pneumonia (the death rate from all-cause pneumonia was essentially the same).

"Not significantly reduced"—this is because (as the data clearly indicates) the vaccinated were more likely to die whilst enduring non-pneumococcal pneumonia. This begs the question, "Which of the other disease characteristics are different enough to not be categorised as pneumonic? Were there any significant differences there between the vaccinated and unvaccinated, and if not, what difference was there?" We have a very small window of disease-characteristic observation, but the one very broad window is the mortality data, which, thankfully, is included in this trial. I think this is a good trial, although I wish more disease symptoms were included so we could investigate more ... I also wish it was still going; I would be very interested to see where it's all at nowadays with the mortality rate.

Perhaps the metals included in the vaccine, or some other compounds in the adjuvants, were primarily responsible for affecting the chances that the body would go through with pneumococcal pneumonia. I'd be interested to know what the lung cancer data was, and of course the rest of the disease incidence data, especially by now, 10 years later (what, can't we afford a well-controlled safety and efficacy trial for that long???).

This is the only effectiveness trial I found on this website which included a saline placebo injection... I found another trial on this vaxopedia website that showed microbial strain detection (diagnostic) mitigation, and the placebo ingredients weren't disclosed. There are a few trials with saline-injection placebos monitoring for antibody generation and safety, but no indications that the vaccinated fared better overall in health and/or disease than the unvaccinated.

These safety and immunogenicity (measuring the antibody generation) trials of vaccine vs saline need to go for over two years, in my opinion, measuring all disease symptoms (effectiveness, per se), and with weight-adjusted dosages to account for what the baby human undergoes.

Here is the other trial mentioned a paragraph earlier. I couldn't figure out what was used as the placebo, but I'd bet it was some other vaccine, given the serious adverse events didn't differ between the two groups as they do in the other one's I've found comparing saline to vaccine with the measure of serious and non-serious adverse events (basically, disease incidence):

https://www.ncbi.nlm.nih.gov/pubmed/25018116/ Lancet. 2014 Oct 11;384(9951):1358-65. doi: 10.1016/S0140-6736(14)61060-6. Epub 2014 Jul 10.

Clinical efficacy and safety of a novel tetravalent dengue vaccine in healthy children in Asia: a phase 3, randomised, observer-masked, placebo-controlled trial. Capeding MR1, Tran NH2, Hadinegoro SR3, Ismail HI4, Chotpitayasunondh T5, Chua MN6, Luong CQ2, Rusmil K7, Wirawan DN8, Nallusamy R9, Pitisuttithum P10, Thisyakorn U11, Yoon IK12, van der Vliet D13, Langevin E14, Laot T15, Hutagalung Y16, Frago C16, Boaz M17, Wartel TA16, Tornieporth NG14, Saville M18, Bouckenooghe A16; CYD14 Study Group

Of the previous links: Here, another major experiment takes place—an experiment which demonstrated that if a certain vaccination was injected into the human three times in one year, it could make a certain character (dengue) of the disease's "theoretical signature" less likely to be detected in the human over the one year compared to receiving the placebo injection (which again, I couldn't see the ingredients of, but I'll continue as if it was saline).

What outright advantage does this show? If we assume there is nothing else to the story and have built up a cultural fear of this specific character "dengue", we will cheer for the power of our intervention.

This dengue vaccine trial report did not note other disease characteristics as being worthy of observation. The placebo material used was not disclosed.

> The primary endpoint was achieved with 56·5% (95% CI 43·8-66·4) efficacy. We recorded 647 serious adverse events (402 [62%] in the vaccine group and 245 [38%] in the control group).

All this focus on one kind of particle, lacking omniscience in a *constantly evolving* not-so-black-and-white world, and mandatory vaccination: *these are the times* ...

A Bill Gates Production: Herd Immunity Demonstration

A Cluster-Randomized Effectiveness Trial of Vi Typhoid Vaccine in India

Dipika Sur, M.D., R. Leon Ochiai, M.H.S., Sujit K. Bhattacharya, M.D., Nirmal K. Ganguly, Ph.D., Mohammad Ali, Ph.D., Byomkesh Manna, Ph.D., Shanta Dutta, M.D., Ph.D., Allan Donner, Ph.D., Suman Kanungo, M.B., B.S., D.I.H., Jin Kyung Park, Ph.D., Mahesh K. Puri, M.Sc., Deok Ryun Kim, M.Sc., et al. July 23, 2009 N Engl J Med 2009; 361:335-344

DOI: 10.1056/NEJMoa0807521

https://www.nejm.org/doi/full/10.1056/NEJMoa0807521

This "successful" herd-immunity vaccination trial, which Bill Gates was involved in the production of, is the fruit of Gates' vaccination campaign in India. To assess the benefits of a typhoid vaccine, in a region with over sixty-two thousand people living in clustered populations, the entire population was divided into two groups without group-splitting within any of the population-clusters ('herds'). About 60% of all participants in this trial were vaccinated.

One group—the control group—received the hepatitis A vaccine, and the other received the new typhoid vaccine, which resulted in about nineteen thousand vaccinated people each side (60% coverage for each group). All the population clusters/herds of the sixty-two thousand humans contained either hepatitis-A- or typhoid- vaccinated members, to assess the factor of herd immunity (to see how well the unvaccinated members of each group fared against typhoid disease).

The essential reasoning as to why some of the population clusters were vaccinated for hepA, is to stop the placebo effect affecting members of the population clusters that are being compared. We can't have one cluster knowing they have received the typhoid vaccine, and we can't have the professionals making the observations and recordkeeping throughout the trial know which people have received the typhoid vaccine—in order to be "double-blinded"—which is what you want for these kinds of trials. Because the trial focused on typhoid diagnoses, a hepA vaccine that had been proven safe (enough) was used as the placebo control.

In these "effectiveness" trials, what is most often looked at—what is looked at here in this Bill Gates trial—is the targeted diagnosis, which involves a PCR test most of the time. The only other thing that is looked at is whether or not the vaccinated group had *significantly* more disease incidence; if they didn't, then the vaccine is considered safe enough. And, needless to say, if the vaccinated group had significantly less *PCR positive* results for the targeted microbe, the vaccine could be considered effective.

Here in this trial, we have something rare in that we have X-vaccinated humans who don't know what kind of vaccine they have had (50/50 Y or X), and humans living in the same population cluster who have received neither vaccine, being strictly monitored for X diagnosis (over two years' time).

The data indicates that typhoid-vaccinated members were more likely (insignificantly) to develop typhoid than their unvaccinated herd members living in the same population cluster (the vaccine is still considered a success).

What is successful about this trial—what is cheered about—is that the group of clusters that had the 60% typhoid vaccine coverage had significantly fewer typhoid diagnoses. The hepA vaccinated herds had overall 150% more typhoid, which to me means the chance of a hepA-vaccinated herd member being diagnosed with typhoid is 150% higher than that of the typhoid-vaccinated herd member's chances of being diagnosed with *typhoid* throughout this trial ...

(*Nota bene:* 'Vi' vaccine means typhoid vaccine, the vaccine under trial.)

At baseline, there were 62,756 residents in the 80 trial clusters, of whom 61,280 were eligible, according to age criteria for participation in the trial ... A total of 37,673 subjects were vaccinated: 18,869 in the Vi vaccine group and 18,804 in the hepatitis A vaccine group. During 2 years of follow-up, 2549 vaccinees (7%) died or migrated out of the study area, and 44 vaccinees (0.1%) migrated to another cluster within the study area.

In this trial, the only disease condition reported—other than typhoid—was paratyphoid: 'Paratyphoid fever was diagnosed in 54 subjects in the Vi vaccine group, as compared with 49 subjects in the hepatitis A vaccine group'. The people who had the lowest rate of typhoid fever during this trial were the unvaccinated who lived amongst the typhoid-vaccinated (this suggests herd-immunity alone is stronger than *the vaccination plus herd immunity*, or that this particular typhoid vaccine increases recipients' chance of developing typhoid by 38%). I'm keen to see much more than just paratyphoid diagnoses ... a whole tally of disease incidence should be on display for us to see, but it's as if the scientific spirit of our culture hasn't asked for it yet.

The data from table 4 (table 4 in the NEJM trial report) shows the typhoid statistics: 16 out of 12,206 unvaccinated humans developed typhoid (.13%) from the typhoid-vaccinated herds, and 31 out of 12,877 unvaccinated humans (.24%) developed typhoid in the hepA-vaccinated herds. Furthermore, 50 out of 31,075 humans developed typhoid in the typhoid-vaccinated herd, and 127 out of 31,681 humans developed typhoid in the hepA-vaccinated herd.

From this data, I have refined the numbers of the *vaccinated humans only*, which when compared to their unvaccinated herd members, is most interesting to me:

Typhoid-vaccinated humans: 34 out of 18,869 (.18%) were diagnosed with typhoid. This means a 38% higher rate of typhoid than in unvaccinated humans of the same herd/population clusters.

Hepatitis-A vaccinated: 96 out of 18,804 people (.51%) were diagnosed with typhoid. This means a 108% higher rate of typhoid than their unvaccinated herd members. This comparison of the vaccinated and unvaccinated within the clusters seems just as reliable to me, because two clusters may vary in socioeconomic status, and other significant things may also be unclear (placebo factor trade-off).

> During the first 30 days after vaccination, there were 18 deaths (10 in the Vi vaccine group and 8 in the hepatitis A vaccine group) and 1 nonfatal serious adverse event (subarachnoid hemorrhage in the hepatitis A vaccine group). Eleven deaths were due to cardiovascular causes and one each to diabetes, burns, malaria, poisoning, tuberculosis, and upper gastrointestinal bleeding; the cause of one death was unknown. None of the events were judged to be causally related to vaccination.

If 18 vaccinated people died in 30 days, that's .6 deaths per day, and yet over the two-year period we have an average of 3.5 deaths per day for vaccinated people, suggesting that the 30 days after the vaccination took place was a time (perhaps the colder season) of natural, low-death rates (4.6% of the entire two-year duration) or that vaccination increases the likelihood of the person dying in some kind of way that kicks-in some time after 30 days of being vaccinated. The mortality rate of the unvaccinated are not available for comparison, surely not because Bill Gates couldn't afford to collect it. What we have regarding mortality data is this fact: 2549 vaccinated people died during this two-year trial.

If you look at the Baseline Characteristics (Table 1), you will find slight variations between the two, arguably favouring the Vi clusters, and arguably making for a different overall position for the groups. Maybe these differences indicate a difference in susceptibility, if not only for typhoid specifically. The two groups may have been equally-susceptible to "disease", whilst varying in susceptibility to the typhoid character of disease.

31

It seems we have substantial proof from this trial report that being vaccinated with the particular HepA vaccine used in the trial increases your chances of being diagnosed with typhoid, and that a vaccine can be championed as successful during a trial whereby unvaccinated recipients within the exact same settings (only differing in *conscious vaccination status*) had a lower rate of the targeted diagnosis. Are we supposed to think that the fact the vaccinated people knew they were vaccinated with something made them more likely to develop the diagnosis than their unvaccinated herd members (it happened in both groups...)? Consider that everyone who is vaccinated in real life generally knows about it, and that if a vaccine provides protection, it generally does so first and foremost for the recipient of the vaccine.

In this study, it is written that the average typhoid rate was 1.42 per 1000 people in the trial region the year before the trial occurred: this is my calculated average for the whole population, which you are invited to check—the data is in the trial report I linked a few paragraphs back, which is freely available to us all. For sixty-two thousand people over two years we could expect to see 176 cases of typhoid if the situation stayed the same. Thirty percent of the population was vaccinated against typhoid and another 30% was vaccinated against hepatitis A, and over the two years that passed after this coverage, 177 cases of typhoid were found.

How should we demonstrate *the herd immunity thing*? *Vaccinated vs unvaccinated* relies on the equal randomisation of organisms in each group within a consistent environment, which is as close as we can get, and we can get pretty close in this regard using fully controlled containments for chickens or rats or dogs, with the exact same humidity and temperature levels and all. Paddocks, on the other hand—unless they are two small paddocks tightly packed with cows, side by side (this would be worthwhile too), we would have to rely on two large paddocks of say 100 acres, and even though they are both near each other, they may have different frequencies of wind and temperature and humidity, and yet still it's probably worthwhile, considering what we have. A very simple structure would settle this: vaccinated group vs unvaccinated group, same species and pedigree, 60% coverage, in exactly the same conditions (an environmentally-controlled facility); until then, I am looking for anything close to that, and this Bill Gates trial from India appears as the closest we can get so far, for whatever reason.

The Flu Vaccine

I set out to analyse what controlled experimentation I could find on the kind of vaccine that is most often advertised to us all. I have included the first two successful trials that I could find, which took me several hours of searching on the internet. After harassing some Facebook groups for a successful *controlled flu-vaccine trial*, I was told to search on *clinicaltrials.gov*, and found that most of the trials I was searching for hadn't had the results published. It seems I found the cream of the crop for flu-vaccine trials. Most trials with published results on this site are comparing one vaccine to another vaccine. I couldn't decide on how to write up the details of each trial; as you can see, they are written quite differently—the way the reference to certain details is written—to the other trials I have referenced … this is because the clinicaltrials.gov website has a unique and inconsistent way of listing all the details, and I am inclined to share the reference details in a similar way to the website.

If our communal friends and health professionals are imploring us to get the flu vaccination, we should at least all see the solid (controlled) science behind why we should. Here is some reasoning protracted from one of the "successful" flu-vax trials that I found:

Phase 3 Trial of Serbian Seasonal Influenza Vaccine (Torlak-300)

Results Point of Contact

Name/Title:Katarina Ilic

Organization:Institute of Virology, Vaccines and Sera, Torlak

Phone:+381 11 3953 700 ext 214

Email:kilic@torlak.rs

Responsible Party: Institute of Virology, Vaccines and Sera, Torlak

ClinicalTrials.gov Identifier:	NCT02935192
	History of Changes
Other Study ID Numbers:	Torlak-300
	VAC 053 (Other Identifier: PATH)
First Submitted:	October 13, 2016
First Posted:	October 17, 2016
Results First Submitted:	June 18, 2018
Results First Posted:	April 19, 2019
Last Update Posted:	April 19, 2019

It seems we, the general people, don't have easy access to these outright assessment trials indicating the overall benefit of the flu vaccine, and that the only two I—an avid searcher of such trials—have found after hours of searching says nothing for flu-vaccine benefits. We are all told by the local pro-vaxxers about the greatness of the flu vaccine and how it is socially imperative to get, as if *it's just obvious* how beneficial it is.

A heap of work resulted in this trial, which included investigating the vaccine-induced change to the serological terrain (the change in the blood compounds, the immunoglobulin/so-called-*antibodies*). It is assumed you want these vaccination-induced antibodies in your blood in high numbers; certain antibodies close-enough to the measured antibodies that are used when you actually have a flu-affected body are involved in the logistical process of unwanted materials: all we can say for certain about *antibody* is that 'antibody/antibodies' pertain to immunoglobulin (no single antibody has ever been isolated): immunoglobulin is employed in the maintenance and reparation of our body: immunoglobulin is measured in the blood as a marker of whether the vaccine worked. Detection of specific antibodies is said to be measured as markers of success, although to me it seems there is no proof of *specifically individual* antibodies. *What definitely is detected is a ramping up of immunoglobulin*, along with some reactions to materials (primers) idealised to be pertinent and exclusive only to the idealised antibodies (detection methods / tools that I doubt have been properly calibrated/controlled for such specificity). The specific-antibody idea goes hand-in-hand with the vaccination idea, otherwise we'd just have one vaccine to boost our immunoglobulin—in a special way that nature doesn't—and be done with it.

Antibody theory digression

This is an excerpt from my friend's article (found at his website https://viroliegy.com/2022/10/31/the-chemical-structure-of-antibodies/), he has done the work of analysing the whole history of *antibody theory*: 'In order to break down and identify the chemical structure of an antibody, logic would dictate that an antibody, like "viruses," would need to be properly purified and isolated from everything else and shown to actually exist first. However, from 1890 when antibodies were initially dreamt up in the mind of Emil Von Behring on up to this point in 1961 when it was decided that these entities were chemically defined structurally by two different researchers, antibodies had never been seen. They were (and still are) nothing more than hypothetical constructs based off of the results from grotesque animal and chemistry experiments which are used to explain the theoretical concept of immunity.' I cannot find a single photo of a whole antibody (non CGI).

Let's grant that there are specific antibodies generated from vaccination which can be used to ward off infections: we should be able to measure this effect if it exists in real-life, using controlled experimentation (science). It seems no team of humans has specifically demonstrated the real-world benefit of having—extra material anyone has called 'antibody'—built-up in your blood. Alas, as a traction-control feature of this book, we shall continue as if we accept fully that there are individual blocks that build up in the blood which we are calling *antibodies,* and *vaccination* can cause your body to produce a heap of *specific antibodies* which only work/remove specific materials from your blood... From what has presently been measured—we can see from plenty of experiments how beneficial this can be in the real world of disease genesis—no one seems to have found an experiment where there was any overall benefit demonstrated for *artificial antibody generation* (vaccination).

Back on track

Perhaps when you have the flu, your body is dealing with heightened *loads* of immunoglobulin and 'viruses' as a part of a refurbishment process. Perhaps what people call 'viruses' are cellular waste and debris being dumped in a dynamic expulsion or reparation/renovation. After vaccination you often don't develop a flu-like disease, but you do produce a heap of immunoglobulin in response to the vaccine injection, and this is cheered-about and highlighted in this clinical trial. The genesis of the extra immunoglobulin—said to be the generation of *specific antibodies*—is the vaccination's best show for itself. And again, I haven't seen the outright benefit scientifically demonstrated in having this concentrated specific-antibody/immunoglobulin terrain induced (perhaps if one is being injected with a large and abrupt load of specific antigens (e.g., *vaccinated*). Perhaps the altered serological terrain—or bio-chemical evolution that follows from this—can meddle with the PCR testing process and change the chances in general that someone will pass as positive or negative for *this* or *that* microbe within the usual detection parameters for PCR.

As I analyse the data of disease incidence in this trial, it appears to me that the placebo group arguably fared better than the vaccine group, as demonstrated in the following results:

Adverse events (the higher the percentage the worse it is): vaccine group scored 4.17%; saline placebo group scored 5.13%. *Serious adverse events:* vaccine group scored .64%, saline placebo scored 0%. No mortalities. It looks like this one ran for 90 days of disease incidence monitoring.

https://clinicaltrials.gov/ct2/show/results/NCT02935192?cond=Influenza&rank=24&view=results

Another flu vaccine trial, the second one I found:

A Randomised, Double-blind, Placebo-controlled Phase IIb Trial to Test FLU-v Vaccine

Sponsor:

PepTcell Limited

Collaborators:

Seventh Framework Programme

University of Groningen

University Medical Center Groningen

Robert Koch Institut

Norwegian Institute of Public Health

Information provided by (Responsible Party):

Here is another trial, this time comparing four different groups of humans that were injected at the start of the trial and then 21 days later, monitored for 4 months of what is considered to be flu season. The 4 comparative groups were established like this:

Full-vaxxed: flu vaccine on both days 0 and 21

Semi-vaxxed: flu vaccine on day 0 and saline on day 21

Saline: placebo on days 0 and 21

Adjuvanted: placebo (no flu vaccine, only the adjuvants of it) on day 0 and   saline placebo on day 21

It is interesting to see how each group differed in the adverse events and PCR test results. The various concoctions of injection that each group received seems to have changed the outcome in different ways. Chemically altering the body will change the likely outcome of physiological and biochemical characteristics, and corollary markers. In this trial, there was no overall advantage for the vaccinated. The humans who received the influenza vaccine were significantly less likely to pass positive for the targeted PCR result (which means a lowering of the targeted diagnosis). This, along with the following information, means it has been scrutinised by our culture as a successful vaccine (i.e. it's safe enough):

Adverse events: group 1 scodred 70.69%, group 2 scored 87.72%, group 3 scored 84.38%, and group 4 scored 88.89%. Serious adverse events: group 1 scored 3.45%, group 2 scored 3.51%, group 3 and 4 scored 0%. No mortalities.

(https://clinicaltrials.gov/ct2/show/results/NCT02962908?view=results)

It looks like this trial went for 42 days of disease incidence monitoring.

Vaccinated adult beagle dogs are compared to "age-matched" unvaccinated adult mystery-breed dogs... and some unvaccinated beagle puppies.

Abdelmagid, Omar & Larson, Laurie & Payne, Laurie & Tubbs, Anna & Wasmoen, Terri & Schultz, Ronald. (2004). Evaluation of the efficacy and duration of immunity of a canine combination vaccine against virulent parvovirus, infectious canine hepatitis virus, and distemper virus experimental challenges. Veterinary therapeutics : research in applied veterinary medicine. 5. 173-86.

https://www.researchgate.net/publication/8150149_Evaluation_of_the_efficacy_and_duration_of_immunity_of_a_canine_combination_vaccine_against_virulent_parvovirus_infectious_canine_hepatitis_virus_and_distemper_virus_experimental_challenges

On three different occasions within two months, dogs were challenged with antigenic injections (three different kinds of antigen).

The vaccinated beagle dogs that were put through this trial were vaccinated four years before, and they grew up together. It seems that the unvaccinated dogs were of a different breed/pedigree and they definitely were from a different facility; the unvaccinated dogs came from two different facilities, whereas the vaccinated were all beagles from the same facility.

> Ten beagle puppies seronegative to CPV-2b, CAAV-1, canine adenovirus type 2 (CAV-2), and CDV were vaccinated at 7 to 8 weeks of age with two doses of vaccine given 3 weeks apart; the puppies were held in isolation until challenge. ... Seven age-matched unvaccinated puppies were held separately at the same facility as controls. Three of the seven controls were entered into the study at the time the other dogs were vaccinated, and the remaining four were introduced 5 months after vaccination. ... An additional three sets of five young beagle puppies

were used as young susceptible controls to validate the virulence of each challenge and are referred to as "young control puppies" in this article.

Perhaps including the 15 beagle puppies in the injection challenges is unnecessary, but *they were beagles.* You might think that this kind of trial would feature 10 vaxxed dogs vs 10 unvaxxed age-matched dogs of the same pedigree from the same facility ... but not here, or anywhere I can find. This is a significant point, to me, because some breeds of dog may be better or worse at dealing with abrupt injections of specific antigens, and different breeds of dogs will grow-up better or worse within specific environmental conditions of upbringing.

There was a clear and significant difference in disease incidence outcomes between the unvaccinated adult dogs and the vaccinated adult dogs, and the puppies. The adult vaccinated beagle dogs were significantly less harmed by the injections.

The science
Imagine this experiment had the same outcomes with proper controls (same breed, age, weight and rearing environment)—let's take it for granted that the lack of weight breed and developmental nurturing is not a significantly confounding factor (as it seems this particular vaccine company is doing, and maybe your local vet). Now, imagine you find a diseased human and you harvest a heap of the materials associated with the disease-process the human is undergoing and inject those materials into another human, and then more humans. Some of them die, but humans with a specifically altered bloodstream extraordinarily loaded with certain fitting antibodies (from and for the advent of vaccination) fare better when you inject these certain materials in their bloodstream. Does this prove the benefit in having that altered bloodstream/immune system in realistic circumstances? This trial is interesting, but even if it was *properly controlled-for* it is not exactly indicative of whether or not you are better off in real-life scenarios having this specifically-altered bloodstream. No organism in real-time is

42

ever introduced to any microbe in the same manner as that which occurred during this trial. To me, this factor alone seems enough to call the experiment unethical.

For the greater good of humanity, why not get 100 dogs (or replace dogs with rats/cows/etc), half vaccinated, and expose them to some contagiously diseased dogs in the enclosure, to trial them in circumstances of real-life disease genesis and witness the advantage or disadvantage of the vaccinated body in disease incidence (even without the sick-dog featuring in the enclosure/containment...)? Here, instead of giving the dogs a chance to show us real-time benefits or detriments of vaccination, we inject them with a heap of disease-associated materials that we harvested (and have a very detailed story about), and we are uncertain of precisely why and how these materials feature in the disease process. What if we ran a trial featuring vaccinated Amazonian Indians versus unvaccinated random humans *who were specifically the same age*, and we neglected to report on their weight and height and developmental environment (which differed), but we included some unvaccinated five-year-old Amazonian Indians ... surely this would be considered insane when we can compare vaccinated humans to unvaccinated humans reared under the exact same conditions and monitored equally, and of the same pedigree/race/strain ... and if we can use saline placebo injections for humans, or, just use animals that don't generate placebo responses to medical ideas, (e.g. "I believe the medicine will save my life" leads to a general increase in healthiness, and so it is on the contrary, the 'nocebo' effect, both have been well and truly measured (*apparently*)) although I wouldn't be crossed if someone did a saline injection on an animal to account for the extraordinary shock the animals experience when being injected (which may be mostly negligible for humans who pre-cognize the process etc etc); on this note, I would like to see some human vaccine trials that lack placebo controls, as this might even cut closer to the reality for humans (excepting *babies*). My ultimate vaccination-experiment prescription for humanity, is outlined in the chapter after this very next one.

Of the five fresh, unvaccinated puppies that were included in each challenge—15 all up—half of them died, probably half of which were euthanised; the details remain unclear regarding the euthanasia thereof.

Anomalies
Throughout this challenge, only one of the adult dogs (unvaccinated) was recorded as having a fever (high rectal temperature). All three of these challenge viruses have as a primary symptom of their associated disease "fever"; even though many became ill, one produced fever and two died—one was euthanised.

One of the most notoriously-thought killers of dogs is 'parvo', which is said to be caused by acquiring the associated particle (virus). For one of dogs' deadliest particles to be given such a helping hand in landing inside the body of a dog (down the nose) as one large army, and not kill any of the dogs, something about the way we are convinced the parvo disease develops seems to be off...

Adeno1 was injected into one of their veins. The only (unvaccinated) adult dog that died from this challenge was euthanised. If we didn't euthanise this one dog and it ended up healing, that would mean out of the parvo and adeno1 virus challenges, none of them managed to successfully overthrow the dogs by themselves, which doesn't sound right given there were likely well into the millions or billions of the virus in both the intravenous insertion and orinasal.

The only dogs that died without being euthanised in the challenge were the dogs that were challenged with the distemper virus both orinasally and intravenously, and they were the same dogs that were orinasally challenged with the parvo virus 28 days before this challenge—two out of four of them died. PhD virologist and molecular biologist Stefan Lanka interprets disease-associated 'viruses' to be the result of cellular degeneration/refurbishing rather than *viral reproduction*; he is one of the more famous academics in the relative field who agrees with my interpretation of the empirical observations on the genesis of microbial diseases (infamous circa 2020); as for the virus-delusion thing, I would bet that he is on the money with that too (he has convinced me personally)... See Germ Theory for more on this.

Here are some excerpts from this dog-injection trial:

> Although serologic response is a good correlate of protection for each of these three antigens, extraneous virus exposure to these agents is likely to occur in dogs in the field, thereby compromising findings.

> The modified-live CPV-2b, CDV, and CAV-2 fractions in the multivalent vaccine evaluated in this study induced immunity in 7- to 8-week-old susceptible puppies that persisted for more than 4 years after vaccination.

Thoughts
I will put some work in for the 'germs-cause-disease' and 'viruses are self-replicated' theories here in this paragraph: If you are worried your dog will die from parvo particle/virus, or any of these notorious so-called microbial particles/viruses like Adeno1, consider that firstly your dog would have to fail at containing the infestation on a small scale wherever/whenever the microbe first begins successfully infecting/reproducing-in a cell of your dog, the virus will grow exponentially from here infecting more and more cells through its progeny/offspring/descendants and the dog would have unfortunately failed at containing the microbe before it successfully reproduced in a dog cell: the four unvaccinated dogs had a large amount / a whole army *suddenly* inserted down their nose—more concentrated introduction frequency than any dog in nature would come close to experiencing—and they managed to sort it out and survive the challenge ... When a dog dies from a naturally developed parvo disease, it assumedly has had the primary issue of developing and/or coordinating appropriate antibodies for the circumstance with single viruses infecting cells and leaving a heap of *slightly varying* offspring. It seems that the real issue, from a germ-

theory point of view, is that at times, dogs can't manage to get the fitting antibodies in to grab the newborn viruses in time before they infect another cell—either the antibodies aren't moving around properly for whatever reason, or they're not attaching to the new viruses properly, or they're not able to be made at all at the time and none of the existing ones will latch onto the incoming viruses that are pouring out of the cells they reproduce in ... And again, *remember*, viruses are theoretically subjected to creative mutations when they reproduce, *in any direction*. We really ought to see some long-term studies in *circumstances of real-life disease genesis* to clear this up.

I've said this before throughout this book: *No healthy human, or animal, has been made ill with a so-called disease-causing microbe through a controlled experiment in a manner that is consistent with real-world circumstances.* If it were achievable, the trial mentioned here would have changed the challenge to the presence of a live, parvo-diseased dog, rather than injecting the cultivated bio-concoction intravenously and/or intranasally...

None of the trials that inject animals with a microbe to see how dangerous the microbe is feature a control microbe: when organisms are killed by adding the microbes that are the theoretical cause of a disease for the organism, the control group doesn't get another kind of microbe or protein/fat/acid parcel of a similar constitution introduced in the exact same manner, which would control for the interactive effect of chemical/physical packages within the environment and even *pressing* upon the organism. All I have ever found is that—if there has been some harm caused to the organism—the microbe was introduced to the organism in an extraordinary manner which compromised the *frequency* of contact, *mode* of contact and/or *concentration* of the microbe/particle. For example, within the part of this book titled Frog Apocalypse I've analysed an experiment that pronounced a clear-cut microbe-alone introduction and difference in mortality for the microbe-introduced–frogs and the frogs who didn't meet the microbe. The frogs who met the microbe had over 8000 zoospores (live, microbial spores that move) per ml, and they were in direct contact with this concoction the whole time—the zoospores were replaced throughout the 30 days to keep them alive. We should include some other zoospores to the control group so that we can control the confounding factor of having permanent contact with such a biomass of live/electric zoospores under the experimental conditions.

Jenner's Tips

'Convictions are more dangerous foes of truth than lies.'

—Friedreich Nietzsche

What did Edward Jenner do?
Edward Jenner made the first vaccine for a notorious disease-character which, in the last thirty years of its existence, has been diagnosed only if a certain marker has been met within a certain detection process. This diagnostic revolution occurred with many disease characters at around the same time. Some similar-looking conditions—like chickenpox, roseola and rubeola (and many others)—acquired this new diagnostic criterion of *particle detection* at around the same time.

The so-called father of modern medicine: in his work "Modern Medicine" (William Osler MD quoting WT Councilman MD; Modern Medicine, Volume 1 p853 Quoted in "The Facts Against Compulsory Vaccination" by R.B. Anderson http:// www.vaclib.org/books/archive1/facts/facts_sm.htm p79): he listed as *the first thing to consider when differentiating smallpox from chickenpox*: "The vaccinal condition of the patient." One more example of the influence that vaccination status has had on the diagnosis of smallpox, can be found in the following, from the "Illinois Medical Journal" in 1923 (Archibald L. Hoyne MD. Smallpox — Its Differential Diagnosis; Illinois Medical Journal, June, 1923 Quoted in "The Facts Against Compulsory Vaccination" by R.B.Anderson http://www.vaclib.org/books/archive1/facts/facts_sm.htm p79): "In examining a case of suspected smallpox, close observation is of the utmost importance. If the patient shows evidence of a typical vaccination scar of comparatively recent date, variola* may be almost absolutely ruled out. (smallpox was commonly referred to as "variola")

Edward's original prophecy was fulfilled as smallpox was no longer diagnosed worldwide within 30 years of the diagnostic revolution; notably, the vaccine had, by this point, been around for nearly 200 years. Jenner successfully transformed a practice originating from the peculiar behaviour of humans into a practice most people circa 2020 are calling *scientific*.

Tip from John Hunter

Edward Jenner is credited with an observation of the animal kingdom that there is a certain bird which lays its eggs in the nest of a foreign bird species; this bird's eggs hatch early and tip the legitimate eggs out of the nest. The parents who have built the nest are tricked into thinking that what hatches from the eggs is their offspring, and proceed to nurture the chicks until they are big enough to fly away (even when the cuckoo begins to look bizarrely different-to—twice the size-of—the unconsciously-fostering nest-building bird). This parasitising bird is called the "cuckoo". Jenner is credited with observing that it isn't the parent cuckoo that tips the eggs out of the nest—it is the freshly hatched baby cuckoo. Jenner was set onto this well before he vaccinated children, by his old teacher, John Hunter. John Hunter and Joseph Banks were intimate friends of Edward's—the same Joseph Banks who received Australian Aboriginal Pemulwuy's skull, and seems to have lost it between himself and the Hunterian Museum in London ... some say his skull was lost in WW2 ... anyway... Joseph Banks at one stage was the president of the Royal Society, also at some stage after becoming president, Joseph swore Edward into the Royal Society, at Edward's request. John Hunter kept a dialogue with Edward after teaching him how to be a physician, and set him onto *the cuckoo mystery*. Edward took some years to come back with a paper on the cuckoo, but when he did, he produced a paper that examined the bird in significant detail... this would have given him the confidence to personally request to be a member of the Royal Society. When Edward was promoting his idea of cowpox insertions to ward against smallpox, he told a large number of veterinarians who disagreed with him—learned people—that they were all *basically wrong*, and that he had figured it out.

Arguing about the origins of the vaccination idea, whether there were legitimate reasons for the idea to take off, is not as useful as looking at the question the same way we ought to have always, today: what have we meticulously recorded in controlled observations/experiments? Alfred R. Wallace, one of the most towering scientific figures of our time, wrote at the end of the fourth paragraph in his first chapter of "Vaccination a Delusion":

> This brief statement of the early history of vaccination has been introduced here in order to give what seems to be a probable explanation of the remarkable fact that a large portion of the medical profession accepted, as proved, that vaccination protected against a subsequent inoculation of small-pox, when in reality there was no such proof, as the subsequent history of small-pox epidemics has shown. The medical and other members of the Royal Commission could not realize the possibility of such a failure to get at the truth. Again and again they asked the witnesses above referred to to explain how it was possible that so many educated specialists could be thus deceived. They overlooked the fact that a century ago was, as regards the majority of the medical profession, a pre-scientific age; and nothing proves this more clearly than the absence of any systematic "control" experiments, and the extreme haste with which some of the heads of the profession expressed their belief in the lifelong protection against small-pox afforded by vaccination, only four years after the discovery had been first announced. This testimony caused Parliament to vote Jenner £10,000 in 1802.

Tip from 'God'

It seems Jenner must have made the empirical observation from a series of small-numbered experiments that if you insert some cowpox-scabs inside some kids' bodies, a mild form of illness will likely manifest (one boy got sick for nine days), and when you do it again (insert pox scabs, from a similar kinds of cellular disease process, *mammalian pox*) two weeks after, *when the child has recovered*, there is likely to be less disease-incidence produced by the child (i.e. the child is less likely to develop a fever). This was a small-numbered experiment done in circumstances inconsistent with the reality of disease genesis, and it's why a whole culture adopted vaccination into its military.

If someone produced fever within several days after having a certain amount of another human's "smallpox" excrement inserted under their skin (*inoculated*), they were considered to have *caught* the smallpox... If someone didn't produce fever when inoculated with smallpox a week or two after having produced fever on being injected with highly-antigenic material (cowpox), we should be sure that this isn't chance and that the dosage levels for inoculation were consistent in the experiments, and even then—Charles Creighton, explained ahead, would agree—this doesn't equate to *vaccine talent*. Edward's experiments were neither well-controlled, nor large-numbered—if in well controlled and large numbered conditions of experiment we find that *being injected with cowpox two weeks earlier than smallpox lowers the chances one will undergo fever after the smallpox injection*, this could be due to the bio-chemical alteration *hangover* within the timeframe following the first antigenic injection. It is possible that the body struggles to deal with a poisoning issue—*in a manner that it ought to*—due to already being tied-up processing some other poisoning issue. People think in terms of disease intensity as to how bad a poisoning affects them, but the failure to extricate some toxins from the body—through intensive distasteful/painful processes—may cause more *overall* significant drawn-out detrimental effects than the short term of fever. The fever may in some cases be the body's *afforded* decision, rather than its *untamed procedure*: **Charles Creighton**, so-called father of modern epidemiology and big so-called *germ theory denier*, published in his book, *Jenner and Vaccination: A Strange Chapter of Medical History* (pp. 149–150):

Jenner himself, in the section of the *Inquiry* where he specifies the sorts of persons for whom cowpox was best suited, mentions a class of children who were apt to resist the inoculation of smallpox altogether. Scrofulous children, with clogged absorbent glands, were of that kind; and his own show case, James Phipps, was a good instance. A large proportion of the variolous tests [the insertion/injection of smallpox excrement underneath the skin], especially abroad, were done upon the inmates of orphanages and foundling hospitals, who are notoriously subject to chronic swelling of the lymphatic glands.

But the most obvious consideration, which should have been familiar to those who first tried cowpox and tested it, was that the vaccine infection itself caused a swelling and obstruction of the absorbent glands in the armpit and neck, and to that extent made them incapable for the time, and in some cases for long after, of taking up and passing into the lymphatic circulation another virus inoculated under the skin at the same place. It was in Paris that this point was chiefly urged by the critics of the variolous test, and the point was at length conceded.

Jenner's tip also could have been produced by a form of *desensitisation* that Jenner mistook for *defensive intelligence*—perhaps the body builds a *chemical callous* in case it is met again with this abrupt-insertion of antigens (which never occurs in nature). Perhaps this is the body's way of preparing for whatever is in its environment, which, for these children, included random abrupt/extraordinarily-large insertions of antigenic material. PERHAPS: When the body has just been injected with filth, it is left with semi-temporary arrangements for *if that happens again in the near future*. If it decides it's worth it, it will adjust the immunological-terrain to cater for this event happening again. What could have effected Jenner's big tip here is what I shall here call the *bodily-bin analogy*: the child's metaphorical–bio-bin was— being average—half-full, and an injection of antigenic material overloaded the bin, prompting a throw-out (through dis- easeful processes), and once the bin was fully emptied— featuring a fever etc—two weeks later, when the child received the next injection of antigenic material, the bin was empty enough to absorb it all without prompting a throw-out (no disease/fever needed). Imagine the metaphorical bin function is orchestrated by cells, and when those cells reach their energy expiry (or have been *crimped* due to some extraordinary occurrence) they will need to be refurbished/recycled/replaced. Imagine inserting such a load of antigenic filth takes up >50% of the child's bin cells' energy quotient to deal with that extraordinary event ... most bodies will be prompted into a full bin recycling on the first, and not on the second after 2 weeks from the first (in this idea/hypothesis/theory). A large-numbered well-controlled experiment, could well elucidate this nebula.

My Proposed Experimental Design

Overview: A proposal to settle, via experiment, the persistently controversial question: "Can vaccination save lives?"—as we appear to lack even one well-controlled experiment demonstrating the widely-accepted lifesaving effect of vaccination, for any species.

Method: 1000 healthy dogs, composed of 500 puppies (<6months old) and 500 adults (>4yo).

The dogs will be divided into two groups/branches, each containing 500 dogs matched for age, weight, height, breed and constitution, differing only in their vaccination status. The trial will have two distinct branches containing 500 dogs (mixed age and vaccination status) each.

- Branch A: 500 dogs (vaxxed and unvaxxed) in the same facility, with same trainers and testers etc.

- Branch B: 500 dogs contained in two separate facilities, vaxxed vs unvaxxed, alternating facilities weekly (swapping).

Facility 1 will hold the 500 dogs in Branch A

Vaccinated: 125 adults and 125 puppies

Unvaccinated: 125 adults and 125 puppies

Structurally identical facilities 2 and 3 will house the two Branch B groups, alternating weekly, each with:

Vaccinated: 125 adults and 125 puppies

Unvaccinated: 125 adults and 125 puppies

54

In summary, half of the 1000 dogs will be vaccinated and half not vaccinated. Five hundred will commence the trial as puppies, and the other 500 as adult four-year-old dogs. The trial will run for three years. The facilities/kennels will all have the same environmental conditions as far as humidity, temperature, lighting, nutriment, air/oxygen flow, and etc goes...

A team of experts will be established to measure the parameters of each individual dog, and a database with each dog's height, weight, age, breed and overall constitution will be established. Of the 1000 individual data entries (dogs), a 50/50 split will be designated with the utmost attention to detail so that we may have two equally composed groups matched for age, weight, height, breed and constitution.

Once the two equally composed groups are established, a 50/50 random-outcome generator (coin flip) will determine the allocation of each (vaxxed or unvaxxed), and vaccination will commence thereafter. Only a select few sworn-in people will have access to the data showing which dogs are vaccinated and which dogs aren't. Nobody involved with the handling/training/measuring of the dogs will have this knowledge (observer-masked).

Dogs are to be monitored daily for signs and symptoms of disease, documenting/reporting thereon.

Dogs are to have their blood measured fortnightly for vital nutrient levels etc., and these are to be recorded in the database.

Dogs (including the pups) will be physically and mentally trained and tested on most days; every dog must receive professional training and testing within every 4-day period during the trial. A performance record will be maintained throughout the trial.

Any signs of disease will be dealt-to with the utmost care. Dogs recognised during training or kennel-time to be unfit for testing/training will be excluded from the training and testing exercises. Depending on the severity of disease, a dog may be removed altogether from its facility for hospitalisation and/or isolation if dogs become unwell and/or violently unsocial during the trial. Dogs found to have microbial infection are not to be removed solely as a result thereof. The physiological state alone of the dog is to be the determining factor as to whether hospitalisation treatment is appropriate (isolation will be appropriate for dogs that become violently unsocial during the trial, and from-a-distance training and exercising (potentially even euthanasia), will be meted out to these kinds of dogs, and this will be a part of the overall performance record.

All disease-related treatment and phenomena will be meticulously recorded.

At the end of the trial, we will see a comparative score for:

Health/vitality

— Cognitive learning abilities
— Physical prowess
— Social wellbeing
— Blood record-keeping (nutrient levels etc.)

Disease incidence

— An outright measure of perceived disease incidence / physiological adversity (including mortality rates)
— An elaborate database of all the different genres/kinds of disease incidence

If such an experiment seems too complex and strange for the politicians, then I propose a simpler model to cut straight to the point: "Can vaccination lower mortality?" This would involve establishing a herd of 2000 cows, dividing the herd into two equally composed groups with respect to age, breed, height, weight etc. One group would be given all the vaccines recommended for cows, while the other group would remain unvaccinated. This information would not be disclosed until the end of the trial. No one involved in the measuring or handling of the cows throughout the trial should know which ones have been vaccinated and which ones have not. If we can show it is consistently or significantly indicated that the vaccinated are better off in health and disease (in mortality), I'll become a vaccination salesman as I'm convinced that's precisely *the kind of evidence/proof I'd need* to tell people the technique saves lives, otherwise I wouldn't even be able to convince myself of such an effect, given it could be pronounced in well-controlled experimental settings and yet this hasn't been demonstrated.

And an experiment to clearly show the effect of disease contagion is due ... see Germ Theory for more on this part of the puzzle. I'm betting you will not find an experiment that showed the introduction of a theoretically-contagious organism alone caused disease. You will only find extraordinary conditions established—in experiment, conditions well beyond the confines of reality—where *some people* will wager that contagion has been well pronounced. I think ocean animals and trees would be suitable test subjects for this kind of experimentation, as I imagine it would be easier to simulate controlled microbial introduction experiments consistent with real-life parameters such as microbial-concentration (e.g: ppm in a fish tank), mode-of-contact (suspended in cycled water), and *exposure time*.

The Diagnostic Paradigm

Vaccines have demonstrated the ability to discourage the occupation of specific bacteria that have been observed to feature in disease processes. In this trial, (Osman Abdullahi, Angela Karani, Caroline C. Tigoi, Daisy Mugo, Stella Kungu, Eva Wanjiru, Jane Jomo, Robert Musyimi, Marc Lipsitch, J. Anthony G. Scott, Rates of Acquisition and Clearance of Pneumococcal Serotypes in the Nasopharynges of Children in Kilifi District, Kenya, The Journal of Infectious Diseases, Volume 206, Issue 7, 1 October 2012, Pages 1020–1029, https://doi.org/10.1093/infdis/jis447) it is demonstrated that vaccination discouraged the occupation of a strain of pneumococci bacteria. The belief that this bacterium strain is responsible for developing a disease is taken for granted as the report gives the impression that nothing else is worth considering. How we come to blame a germ strain for disease in this modern-day setting is explained in this part, headlined "The most complex of sentences" a few paragraphs away (after "The Party Analogy"). Even if successfully stopping the targeted microbe also successfully stops specific disease characteristics from manifesting, we really ought to be sure we aren't trading disease characteristics/genres for something worse or equal, especially when we know not all reactions/responses/effects play out immediately and tangibly/visibly.

The Party Analogy

Featuring Big Mick
The way we think of disease mitigation could be described like this:

Imagine we hear of parties that feature a certain character/person. During really tragic times—when the party is terrible and people get hurt and/or die—this *one character* (Mick) is often found amongst the drama (a microbe strain).

After many parties ending in tragedy, and as a community recognising they generally always featured Mick, we develop a conviction and Mick gets blamed; fearing that Mick will feature at the next party and cause tragedy, we start to focus on devising things that could discourage him from attending.

We find certain ingredients to add to the party, running a trial comparing parties with these ingredients and parties without to report back that we've found the right ingredients—"we need to include fireworks and bonfires, and then *this bad character called* Mick is consistently significantly-less-likely to show up"—without mentioning the frequency of tragedy, just that Mick is less likely to come along. We declare that we have found a brilliant solution to the problematic parties because originally, before running the trials, we all got together and convicted Mick as the cause of the tragedies he features in. We do this without making a thorough, in-depth analysis of whether *during the trials* the parties with bonfires and fireworks were any more or less likely to feature problems/negative dramas, and people are ignored when they try to tell people "the profile of characters and how they feel together is likely to change for better or worse, and our fear and blaming of Mick has caused a tunnel-vision". We know problems still occur at these parties, yet we feel good about managing to discourage Mick because we all blamed him for being the cause of past problems.

It may turn out that Mick is significantly less likely to attend parties with bonfires and fireworks and they really are less likely to erupt with dramas, fights, etc. at any moment (no vaccine trial I've found has indicated this, metaphorically speaking). If so, in a one-month trial, it might appear to be a great idea to have bonfires and fireworks at all parties as is indicated in the trials to make for a 30% decrease in the chances of a "negative drama" erupting at any moment. Although, unbeknownst to us or the investigators, when drama does occur at parties with bonfires and fireworks, although it may be 30% less likely, it may be 100% more chaotic when it does erupt. Perhaps a more pernicious character wreaks havoc whilst we gloat about our anti-Mick campaign.

We ought to run the trial for at least one year to clear up whether or not we traded a 30% less likely tragedy at any given moment for a 100% increase in chaos and damage when the tragedy does occur. Ten years is probably a good timeframe for this, especially if we are going to force people to have the bonfires and fireworks at their party.

A metaphor that could round this whole exposé off might be this:

We find workers on a building that once was without blemishes, and we blame the workers for the fact that it is in need of reparation. We run experiments and find that a lot of buildings will be set back into a workable mode again if we spray anti-worker on the job sites. The spray will prompt the workers to go away so people can use the building's facilities again, but sometimes this doesn't work to prompt a cessation of the workers and sometimes they end up demolishing the whole thing. Buildings generally need regular upkeep— periodical reparations involving shutdowns of certain facilities or capacities—and workers (including demolition agents). We should be sure that when we spray the workers with anti-worker, we aren't *decreasing the chances of the building completing reparation*, and/or it may not repair/finish as well as it could have if the workers weren't poisoned and hurried-off during the operation.

In this trial (Jennifer R. Scott, Eugene V. Millar, Marc Lipsitch, Lawrence H. Moulton, Robert Weatherholtz, Mindy J. Perilla, Delois M. Jackson, Bernard Beall, Mariddie J. Craig, Raymond Reid, Mathuram Santosham, Katherine L. O'Brien, Impact of More Than a Decade of Pneumococcal Conjugate Vaccine Use on Carriage and Invasive Potential in Native American Communities, *The Journal of Infectious Diseases*, Volume 205, Issue 2, 15 January 2012, Pages 280–288, https://doi.org/10.1093/infdis/jir730), some humans were monitored over 10 years to find that as one bacterium strain (pneumococci) was cleared from the human, a different strain took up the position, and no benefit was demonstrated in terms of health/illness. Technically, the vaccine appears to be working in this case as it lowered a commonly-feared diagnosis involving the presence of the targeted microbe strain.

The most complex of sentences
Point: Theoretically, a potentially infinite amount of different microbe species/forms/strains can manifest. Many different kinds have been profiled so far. Microbes play various roles in bodily processes, including disease. Are microbes the "primary cause" of the processes they play an essential part in? This section looks at the seemingly circular reasoning that supports this notion of blaming the germ. Just because a particular process does not ensue without a particular part (microbe) does not mean that part is the primary cause of the process. A sprocket is not the primary cause of the moving motorcycle.

Some studies appear to provide the rationale for us to embark on a campaign to eradicate certain microbes after deeming them the cause of the disease process they feature in. The following is an account of one of these studies, titled "The fundamental link between pneumococcal carriage and disease": (Birgit Simell, Kari Auranen, Helena Käyhty, David Goldblatt, Ron Dagan, Katherine L O'Brien & for the Pneumococcal Carriage Group (PneumoCarr) (2012) The fundamental link between pneumococcal carriage and disease, Expert Review of Vaccines, 11:7, 841-855, DOI: 10.1586/erv.12.53).

Link to study:
https://www.tandfonline.com/doi/full/10.1586/erv.12.53

The authors claim that vaccine efficacy against disease depends on vaccine efficacy against microbe acquisition and suggest that we can measure a vaccine's potential to prevent illness by measuring its ability to prevent the acquisition of a specific microbe strain. Their study outlines how we come to blame the pneumococci bacteria for two different disease processes in which they feature: Acute Otitis Media (AOM) and pneumonia.

In the article, some key observations purport to explain just how the acquisition of these specific bacteria causes disease: Some animals had the culprit bacteria sprayed into their nasal region, others in their lungs. There was no mention of what else was in the spray. In cases like this, I've often found that numerous contaminating materials, often collected from the site the bacteria were harvested from or the medium in which they were cultivated, are included.

The animals that endured this, of course, suffered adverse effects (worse for the lung-sprayed)—somewhat similar to flu-like *symptoms*, as one might expect (respiratory system dramas and middle-ear inflammation). Microbes can be potent chemical packages; respiratory cells and the like are chemically and physically fragile … when the cellular chemistry naturally changes and gives rise to these extraordinarily-present microbes, how can we argue that the microbe is the primary cause of that change? Is it just because we find destroyed cells, and the microbes associated with the process, and we find that we can destroy healthy mammal respiratory cells when we place these microbes on them in sufficient quantity?

It was observed that when people become ill, they start acquiring a greater variety of bacteria. In this case, they acquire some new strains of pneumococci. Many healthy humans were found carrying these new strains in the days immediately preceding illness (*nota bene*: many healthy people carry strep and pneumococci bacteria, to some degree, without developing the illness; despite said microbes being blamed for causing these and other disease processes: the strains change along with the symptoms of the region). Perhaps the cellular terrain began to change in the days preceding the illness, and thus the microbe strains changed, and we are blaming the microbes because it's easier than figuring out why/how (to tell people) the cellular terrain changed in a way that saw the flourishing of different microbe strains than the usual strains present during full-health.

Different microbes feature in different terrains. In keeping with a general law of nature, an organism proliferates only if the environment is suitable. So, in effect, the terrain selects its resident microbes.

Did the respiratory cells degenerate first and call for the bacteria? Or did the bacterium strains simply come along from outside the body and take the lead role, killing healthy respiratory cells? Why was the body susceptible to developing a respiratory infection that required occupying microbes? Why were the cells vulnerable? Perhaps they were no longer compatible or viable. Perhaps it was no longer advantageous or safe to keep them. And perhaps the body orchestrates disease processes with microbes involved, but then we kill the microbes, often stopping the process, cutting it short ... and during our consequent cheering, we don't consider what we've potentially traded: the thwarting of a beneficial refurbishment process for the cessation of temporary discomfort. Of course, sometimes the infestation persists beyond our intervention, and whether we decreased our chances of healing at all might be a mystery until we run a properly-controlled non-myopic trial.

The body proceeds with a disease process and we record it all in bacterial demographics, apparently oblivious to the possibility that our cells have degenerated and become due for undertaking or strenuous refurbishment (involving microbes), not knowing for certain what the primary trigger of disease was or precisely where the bacteria came from (inside or out) and why. And, thus far, we are convinced a culprit microbe colonised the body from without, with no full explanation other than elaborate abstract calculations of why and how cellular structures end up incompatible and susceptible and need to be refurbished—logistics. We seem satisfied that the germ is to blame outright. It was more than 150 years ago that this became a palatable concept in our culture. From supernatural agents to featuring microbes, we haven't changed the essential dynamic of blaming external entities/agents for our internal eruptions (contagion).

How's this for a sentence:

> During the weeks preceding respiratory infection, children with pneumococcal AOM had a significantly lower frequency of carriage specific to the serotype/group causing the disease compared with children of the same age who also carried pneumococci during a respiratory infection, but did not have pneumococcal AOM, thus confirming the role of recent acquisition of the disease-causing serotype.

The strains of pneumococci that are present during a respiratory infection are different from those present during a middle-ear infection. The authors of this study appear to be claiming that this is sufficient evidence to blame each specific strain for the specific disease (that is, for causing each disease process). Without this culprit, we have nothing to blame except the mechanisms of our own cellular machinery (ourselves).

Furthermore: "Notably, in this study, the serotype causing AOM was found in 99% of the simultaneously obtained NP (nasal swabs) samples from the children affected by AOM."

What would happen if we were to somehow eradicate this strain of bacteria? Would another strain take its place when the body presents conditions suitable for infestation by the original (but now eradicated) strain?

Why are some cells compromised in such a manner that they become infested or undertaken? Perhaps they're not worth salvaging. Perhaps their best-before quota is up.

If we could somehow stop the occupation of all disease-associated microbes (let alone just specific ones), avoiding this disease process of cellular undertaking and regeneration, would we succumb to another diseased condition that doesn't involve microbial infestation? Would the susceptible cells mutate and become cancerous, or would the body simply be burdened with second-class, ill-functioning cells, functioning in a subpar manner, which would also lead it to become more susceptible to ill-functioning and disease? It seems a bit far-fetched to consider…

Getting it done:

> Due to the lack of reliable diagnostic methods and the difficulty in obtaining adequate sample for culture from the infection site, identification of the etiologic agents of pneumonia has remained a challenge. This, in turn, may hamper understanding the relationship between pneumococcal carriage and pneumonia. In spite of these diagnostic challenges, in children aged less than 5 years pneumococcus is recognized as the most important cause of bacterial pneumonia.

Here is one more trial where vaccination demonstrates the ability to discourage a certain strain of bacteria from occupying the human (*to a given-detectable extent*), whilst encouraging the heightened occupation of some other strain/species of bacteria. This study compares the efficacy of a new vaccine to an old vaccine (as is often the case in vaccination effectiveness trials) in stopping the acquisition of specific microbes that are, allegedly, solely responsible for causing disease in humans, with no mention of mitigating disease incidence, just some alleged culprits of it (Ron Dagan, Noga Givon-Lavi, Orly Zamir, Merav Sikuler-Cohen, Lior Guy, Jacob Janco, Pablo Yagupsky, Drora Fraser, Reduction of Nasopharyngeal Carriage of Streptococcus pneumoniae after Administration of a 9-Valent Pneumococcal Conjugate Vaccine to Toddlers Attending Day Care Centers, The Journal of Infectious Diseases, Volume 185, Issue 7, 1 April 2002, Pages 927–936, https://doi.org/10.1086/339525).

Polio

We all have felt the dire emotional charge associated with polio—this has been passed on from our great-grandparents and their ancestors. In the mid 20th century, polio was diagnostically married to a said specific particle/virus. Nowadays, not many of us likely to be reading this book have come across someone diagnosed with polio, and we are also unlikely to have known someone who died from any of the other infamous disease characters such as measles or whooping cough. The first idea that makes sense as to why this is the case nowadays is that things changed when we made vaccinations for these diseases. Polio is perhaps the scariest vaccinated disease people can think of, and seemingly has the most impressive track record of diagnostic evolution.

In 1908, some people (Popper and Landsteiner) filtered the spinal fluid from a human that had died with/from polio and injected it into a monkey, and shortly thereafter paralysis ensued. This was one monkey out of many that were being used in experiments to find the polio virus and, notably, became paralysed after the injection, to determine a microbial cause of polio. Because the filter that was used filtered-out bacteria, it was deduced that polio is caused by a virus. It appears as though only one monkey was made fully paralytic out of god-knows-how-many were experimented upon.

In the 1950s, with the aid of the electron microscope, a kind of virus/particle/material found to be associated with paralytic disease was determined and named "polio". Before the end of the 1950s, polio was the diagnosis given to paralytic cases which now—since the '90s—all come under the umbrella of Acute Flaccid Paralysis (AFP). Of the old polio diagnoses pre-1955, most were non-paralytic, as is well-acknowledged in credible medical journals (quoted ahead).

The commonly-held criteria for diagnosing polio has changed significantly since the 1950s, and nowadays if the criteria aren't met—including paralysis duration and "polio-virus isolation", a patient with paralysis will not be diagnosed with polio but any of the myriad of other conditions which fall under the umbrella of AFP. More to follow/reiterate on this ahead...

India declared a polio-free year in 2012 whilst reporting over 60 thousand cases of Acute Flaccid Paralysis, up from 8103 cases of AFP in the year 2000, as is documented on the WHO website (https://extranet.who.int/polis/public/CaseCount.aspx). AFP grew and polio shrunk, and again: AFP is all paralytic, whereas polio cases before the 60s were allegedly predominantly non-paralytic. Paralytic disease itself didn't erupt this quickly, but the tendency for it to be reported to databases such as the WHO increased over time; this is another example of the evolution of the diagnosis, monitoring and reporting of specific characters we believe cause disease. When AFP diagnosing and reporting criteria got implemented, it spread across the world.

You can't rationally compare earlier pre-vaccination polio diagnosis records with the records of later "laboratory-confirmed polio" cases to assess the impact of a vaccination or the trend of paralytic disease per se. The polio vaccination came hand-in-hand with the doctor enforcing a more rigorous case-definition of polio, and I have great proof of this *a few paragraphs away* from the *Australian Medical Journal*. 'To avoid unwarranted criticism of the vaccine', each polio-vaccinated person must fit the criteria of a rigorous polio diagnosis criteria—sounds fair enough, eh?

Global - Polio and Acute Flaccid Paralysis (AFP)

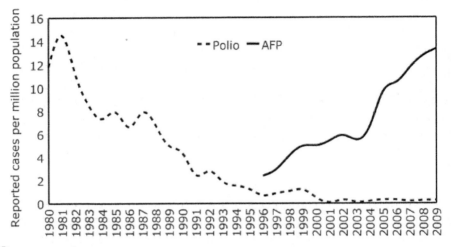

© 2011 Greg Beattie
Sources: WHO for Polio and AFP data
US Census Bureau for population data

Basically, the polio diagnosis today comes under the diagnostic umbrella of AFP and represents only the paralytic kind of polio (the only polio diagnosed these days: the paralytic kind with a specific material-detection result). AFP surveillance began in the 90s, surveying for paralytic disease—not just polio. Paralytic disease is still around and needs to be accounted-for. Paralytic disease surely isn't growing as fast as what the previously-shown graph makes out (if at all), and this is another good point to refer to the fact that notification data is woeful for making any such deductions. As mentioned earlier, before the vaccination came along, a lot of polio was diagnosed for non-paralytic cases, and all was diagnosed without the specific particle-detection result, as is documented in the mainstream literature. Here is an excerpt from the *Medical Journal of Australia*, March 3, 1951, under the heading "The Pathogenesis of Poliomyelittis", just before "laboratory confirmation" (specific particle-detection) of the virus was introduced as a diagnostic criterion:

> It is now known quite well that non-paralytic cases of poliomyelitis far outnumber the paralytic, and indeed it seems reasonable to say that the non-paralytic form of the disease is the normal and typical response of

the human being to the infection, the occurrence of paralysis being unusual and analogous to the occurrence of encephalitis in measles.

Many people were diagnosed with polio if they happened to be feverish and lethargic throughout polio season. Many people would have cashed in on some unwarranted insurance money when they were diagnosed with polio. We will never know what percentage of polio diagnosed before the 1950s would have fit the diagnostic criteria for polio after the 1950s, but it seems we can safely say that most of it wouldn't have, and judging by the statement above, most of it wouldn't be classed as AFP.

The exact data of how and when the diagnostic criteria of polio changed, all the different increments—I don't feel this is necessary to provide beyond the key points of the diagnostic protocol evolution. A thorough investigation of this will lead one to the enlightenment that as polio was being conquered, the diagnostic criteria was tightening, and AFP reports started and began rising rapidly, and the diagnostic machine unconsciously fulfilled the prophecy. And now here we are in 2020 with people calling themselves anti-vaxxers whilst believing the polio vaccine conquered polio (which, to me it kind of did—the vaccine campaign pushed for a more sophisticated diagnostic criteria for "polio", which made the word "polio" occur in diagnosis less frequently).

The *iron lung* thing—that's not around anymore, not because of vaccination but because of positive pressure ventilators: technological advancement (I've been asked by many stout believers in vaccination to explain why I haven't seen a child hooked-up to an iron lung).

From the *Medical Journal of Australia*, June 5, 1952, page 3:

There are many patients who do not develop paralysis in whom the diagnosis of poliomyelitis is suspected, but in the absence of complete laboratory investigation for poliomyelitis, which is not yet available in Australia, an accurate diagnosis is impossible. However, the condition of an ever-increasing number of patients, who at one time would have been regarded as having non-paralytic poliomyelitis, is being more correctly diagnosed by improved laboratory methods.

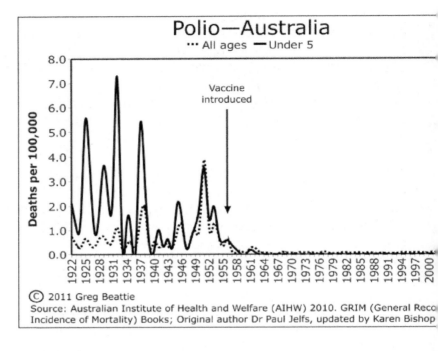

Polio—Australia
··· All ages — Under 5

Vaccine introduced

© 2011 Greg Beattie
Source: Australian Institute of Health and Welfare (AIHW) 2010. GRIM (General Reco Incidence of Mortality) Books; Original author Dr Paul Jelfs, updated by Karen Bishop

Doctors were encouraged by the medical literature to be more discerning in diagnosing polio, and perhaps encouraged by their own personal interests to follow on in this manner so as not to diagnose their patient with what they vaccinated them for: "the vaccine targets the microbe strain; we need to be specific to avoid unwarranted criticism of the vaccine we assured you works" ... Doctors in Australia who received this new polio vaccine of Jonas Salk's (or whoever's) that had been *successfully trialled* for usage one year earlier are very likely to have read this excerpt from the *Medical Journal of Australia*, July 28, 1956, page 158 (bold emphasis is my own):

DIAGNOSTIC CRITERIA FOR POLIOMYELITIS

The diagnosis of poliomyelitis in persons vaccinated against poliomyelitis assumes considerable importance in assessing the degree of protection afforded by the vaccine. Once immunisation commences the public mind will be as in a poliomyelitis epidemic, and such is the fear of the disease, that any illness is likely to be considered to be poliomyelitis until someone in authority says it is not.

It is hoped that the following list of diagnostic criteria will not only help practitioners in what is often a difficult diagnosis, but may **prevent unwarranted criticism of the vaccine** by incorrect notification of poliomyelitis in vaccinated persons; or more important, incorrect provisional diagnosis.

These diagnostic criteria may be divided into three categories:

1. Symptoms and signs usually present in poliomyelitis

2. Symptoms and signs present in other acute infections, but rarely seen in poliomyelitis—the so-called "negative indicators"

3. The symptoms and signs of the paralysis which may occur in poliomyelitis."

Note: the medical literature from 1951 quoted a few paragraphs back that 'It is now known quite well that non-paralytic cases of poliomyelitis far outnumber the paralytic'.

Furthermore, in the same article, after an elaboration of these three aforementioned categories, laboratory confirmation of the vaccinated-against virus strain (specific material-detection) is said to be needed for a precise diagnosis:

Laboratory methods of diagnosis of poliomyelitis: it should be emphasised that in many patients, particularly the non- paralytic type, it is not possible to make a precise diagnosis of poliomyelitis without laboratory confirmation. Even in the presence of a lower motor neuron paralysis, examination of the cerebrospinal fluid may reveal that the condition is due to acute infective polyneuritis, in which condition as a rule there is no increase in cells.

71

The following laboratory methods should be adopted in all cases where any doubt exists: (a) examination of the cerebro-spinal fluid, (b) isolation of poliomyelitis virus, (c) positive serological tests... (d) serological antibody tests to exclude mumps, herpes simplex and other causes of meningo-encephalitis.

More significant diagnostic evolution occurred in the 60s, as I have found proof of in the *Australian Medical Journal* (Poliomyelitis in Australia; Med J of Aust: Nov 4, 1967 861-862): it seems that doctors were no longer permitted to diagnose polio. All suspected cases were to be referred to the Poliomyelitis Surveillance Committee. A panel of experts was established to confirm each diagnosis. This panel, called the Poliomyelitis Surveillance Committee, gave a second and final opinion on cases that were proposed by doctors as still fitting the criteria. In other words, doctors who believed they had a case of polio on their hands had to refer all the evidence to this panel.

And still, more significant evolution of the polio diagnostic criteria occurred. It is very sophisticated nowadays. The current case definition for polio is found here, amongst other places: http://www.health.gov.au/internet/main/publishing.nsf/Content/cda-surveil-nndss-casedefs-cd_polio.htm. To say it is sophisticated and elaborate compared to 1930s polio diagnostic protocol could be an understatement. Along the evolutionary path, many countries were still diagnosing polio the old way, and when vaccination teams swooped in endeavouring to conquer polio in a given region, they brought along and spread their diagnostic evolution—laboratory teams—and vaccinated everyone, then educated practitioners on how to precisely diagnose the disease (and "avoid unwarranted criticism of the vaccine"), only diagnosing polio if they went through the newly instilled diagnostic protocols.

Many different diagnoses fit the old diagnostic-criteria of polio: Chinese Paralytic Syndrome (McKhann et al. Clinical and electrophysiological aspects of acute paralytic disease of children and young adults in northern China; The Lancet: Vol 338; Sept 7, 1991 p593-597 http://www.thelancet.com/journals/lancet/article/PII0140-6736%2891%2990606-P/abstract). Some researchers have had a closer look at the data, with a later study in Hebei Province finding that both this new disorder and the Guillaine-Barre Syndrome *were* really polio. The researchers came to their conclusion after looking at the trends in polio from 1955–1990. It was noted that, after mass vaccination started in 1971, reports of polio went down, but Guillaine-Barre Syndrome increased about ten-fold (Shen et al. What causes Chinese paralytic syndrome?; The Lancet: Vol 344; Oct 8, 1994 p1026 http://www.thelancet.com/journals/lancet/article/PIIS0140-6736(94)91688-8/fulltext).

Here is an excerpt from an article written by the vice-chairman of the Indian Medical Association's Sub-Committee on Immunisation. The article appeared in India's national newspaper, *The Hindu*. It starts with:

> It is now being acknowledged that the National Polio Eradication Programme did not work according to plan. The failure of this magic bullet approach (repeated doses of oral polio vaccine) to solve what is essentially a water and sanitation problem was predictable. Yet, that did not mitigate the sadness its failure caused among many of us who have worked tirelessly to make it succeed. The Indian Medical Association (IMA) Sub-Committee on Immunisation debated on whether to go public with its findings about the failure of this initiative. In August 2006, it concluded that it was its duty to do so.

(The Hindu, Sunday, Nov 19, 2006
http://www.hinduonnet.com/thehindu/
mag/2006/11/19/stories/2006111900100400.htm)

India - Polio and Acute Flaccid Paralysis (AFP)

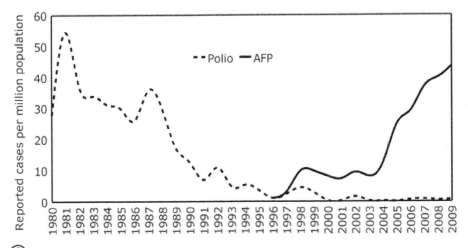

© 2011 Greg Beattie
Sources: WHO for Polio and AFP data
US Census Bureau for population data

There's been a lot said about the now-illegal pesticide DDT causing polio. I found an article from the 40s which provides reason to suggest that DDT caused some of what was diagnosed as polio, but the authors of the article didn't entertain the hypothesis. "The Journal of Pediatrics VOL. 28 JANUARY, 1946 NO. 1 Original Communications epidemic poliomyelitis Lores F. Gebhardt, Ph.D., M.D., and William McKAY, M.D., C.P.H. Salt Lake City, Utah"

Material concocted together and determined to be 'polio virus' could be seen at this stage in the 40s (I think the 'isolating' of the virus must have settled in the 50s), but this kind of detection/isolation/observation wasn't readily accessible, hence doctors didn't diagnose polio according to virus detection until the 50s when things became more developed (including the first licensed polio vaccine). Some people mistake this "DDT caused polio" thing for a claim that all polio is or was caused by DDT. Remember that the concept of "all polio" is not so straightforward, because if you're talking about polio in 1901, or even in the 40s when we could detect the 'virus' material but it rarely occurred for diagnosis, in Australia and America at least, that's a significantly different diagnostic criteria to the polio of 1956. The strongest correlation the investigators of the aforementioned study found when analysing all the potential leads that may have been indicative of a polio virus acquisition hotspot, including people who swam in swimming pools and people who got bitten by insects, by far, was this:

> A combination of the two categories, unwashed or unpeeled fresh fruits and vegetables, shows that 206 out of 206, or 100 per cent, of the patients with poliomyelitis in the survey had eaten these foods one to two weeks or more prior to developing the disease.

I wonder if, back then, it would be extraordinary (statistically significant) for 206 people selected at random from Utah 1950 to all have eaten unwashed or unpeeled fruits or vegetables within two weeks ... this is not a solid reason to think DDT caused polio, although I'd be more inclined to think it was the DDT on the fruit and veg than the theorised *human polio virus* in the animal manure fertiliser deposited on the produce...

From The Medical Journal of Australia, Feb 9, 1952, page 170:

> When a virus infection is initiated in the body of a person with no pre-existing immunity, it is only on the rarest occasions that the virus finds it possible to sweep through and produce serious damage in all or most of the cells that are theoretically susceptible to its action. Much more often the virus has to fight its way through a whole series of obstacles that we are only beginning to particularize—obstacles at the surface of the cell and within the cell, interference phenomena by which a non-virulent virus can block the activity of a virulent one, failure of cells in which virus has multiplied to liberate the new brood of virus particles and so on. None of these processes have yet been clearly defined, but they must be invoked if we are to understand the basis of subclinical infection.

How to turn a disease that is apparently 10 times under-detected and under-reported *worldwide* into a disease that is only six times under-detected and under-reported?

Put in a bigger effort (credible references to this ahead).

Before delving into the recent media measles hype since the measles vaccine was going out of fashion, let's first examine evidence of significant measles diagnostic evolution:

Surveillance of measles in England and Wales: implications of a national saliva testing programme

M. Ramsay,[1] R. Brugha,[2] & D. Brown[3]

The impact of a mass vaccination campaign against measles–rubella in England and Wales was assessed using the results of a saliva test for measles-specific IgM, which was offered to all notified cases of measles. By means of clinical data supplied by the reporting doctors, we estimated the sensitivity and specificity of various clinical case definitions in predicting a confirmed case. A saliva sample was obtained within the appropriate time period for 3442/7574 (45.4%) of notified cases; the proportion confirmed by saliva testing was low and fell from 67/681 (9.8%) at the start of the campaign to 1/373 (0.3%) after 35 weeks. The

When the new test for measles was introduced in the study pictured above, it was found that about 93% of the previous measles patient-samples were not positive for measles under the new measles diagnostic criterion of specifically-alleged microbial-strain/material presence. The measles diagnosis evolved seemingly to avoid unwarranted criticism of vaccination (because vaccination supposedly works against a specific microbe) and perhaps simply to make things more sophisticated, as to more correctly assess the efficacy of the vaccination, we need to diagnose measles based on microbial presence
(https://apps.who.int/iris/bitstream/handle/10665/55295/bulletin_1997_75(6)_515-521.pdf;jsessionid=BEE4A7D6DE984D422C5DFEF0822C4325?seque

nce=1). As I just *basically* said, the disease is nowadays diagnosed only if a specific marker within a specific detection process is met. In the past, this character of disease that we now call measles has featured in major epidemics; most of the diagnoses made of measles have probably been diagnosed according only to clinical symptoms. It is worth noting that the big revolution in diagnostic protocols started occurring around the 1950s.

When a story stating *"vaccination rates have dropped due to antivax propaganda"* gets put out through all the major media outlets, the financial-muscle of the vaccine-producing industry is flexing, and it is quite impressive. A call is put out to many medical practices, journals and media outlets exclusive to medical practitioners by organisations like the CDC and WHO, to start increased surveillance of measles, *be hypervigilant of measles*, send blood samples of ANY suspected case of measles to the lab, even test people who have been vaccinated (*disregarding the diagnostic aid*) because VAX RATES HAVE DROPPED, so we must be on the lookout for this deadly disease as we anticipate its spreading.

From here, doctors become hyper-vigilant, sampling patients for *measles marker detection* (especially if the patient isn't vaccinated against measles) because they're now on the lookout for the deadly virus which the big organisations expect to erupt into plague proportions at any moment, *especially if the clinicians don't find all the measles*. Thus, during this period, we see the notification reports increase quite drastically.

"A spike in measles cases in Australia has prompted immunisation warnings. Are you at risk?"

ABC article 10th of April 2019

(https://www.abc.net.au/news/health/2019-04-10/measles-spikes-prompts-immunisation-warning-are-you-at-risk/10986172?fbclid=IwAR1zauuzNxWGFaZamqCX_SPzyngRP-PfoiWLPzW__zG83qaZMbAyrlehz2A)

"Measles cases quadruple globally in 2019, says UN"

"Vaccination deniers gaining ground"

BBC article 16th of April 2019

https://www.bbc.com/news/health-47940710

More from the BBC article: "Twenty million plus lives since 2000 saved from the vaccine." The article says that numbers of *reported* measles have quadrupled! It also says, "The agency said actual numbers may be far greater since only one in 10 cases globally is reported." No mention is made of the cause of this extraordinary shift in the surveillance and reporting incentive (the percentage of people tested for measles and the frequency of reporting cases). The lacking measles-vaccine uptake and the increased measles-surveillance and news articles, seemingly started from *the vaccine-induced autism media hype*.

Why would such a change in diagnosing, monitoring and or reporting occur?
It's documented in these articles. They say how doctors and surveillance teams are *now gearing up* to see and report every case of measles possible after people have stopped vaccinating due to anti-vax propaganda. These articles admit that there is to be *more testing for measles* and that *more cases are to be reported*. See also: https://www.ausdoc.com.au/views/stand-tall-gps-youre-frontline-renewed-war-measles. I can no longer access this article because I do not have the prerequisite status. Such articles state "doctors are urged to suspect measles in anything, from as much as a rash or fever".

Disease-Featuring Cultural-Devastation

The extent to which the current Germ Theory of disease-causation is cemented in our culture became apparent to me when I read Jarryd Diamond's *Guns, Germs, and Steel*. He explained that microbes evolved alongside humans, which I agree with: as human biology and environment changes, so too will our endogenous (inner) and exogenous (outer) microbial agents within the culture.

Diamond, whilst providing brilliant cutting-edge explanations of many things, noted the diseased states of peoples (generally the indigenous) during the acculturation that occurred in all the European invasions of America, Australia and the Pacific islands, and explains *as a matter of fact* that majority of the indigenous peoples who died of disease died solely because of the *savage germs* riding on the invaders. This is a very big statement when you consider how it is commonly accepted that most of the indigenous population died as a result of European settlement (they lost more than 50% of their original numbers), and it is commonly accepted that most of them died from disease rather than warfare. The European invaders were allegedly immune to these killer microbes, whilst the invaded people weren't. This made me wonder why indigenous peoples didn't have their own army of savage germs, why this microbe war was apparently one-sided, why the invaded people suffered more disease after a successful invasion every time.

Out of all these continents and islands of indigenous peoples that Europeans have made contact with/invaded, why is there no account of any new disease-causing microbes that the Europeans weren't immune-to but which the indigenous people were?

Turns out, we have two excuses in the mainstream doctrines: Europeans bred microbes that could only survive amongst civilisation-sized populations; for instance, measles apparently needs 500 thousand people in one area (F. L. Black,

"Measles endemicity in insular populations: critical community size and its evolutionary implication," Journal of Theoretical Biology 2 [1966]: 207–11), and Europeans bred microbes that came from horses and/or cows. The mainstream literature says living with civilisation microbes has been our strongest selection-pressure/shaping-force.

Why don't we hear of any Aztec microbes ravaging the Spaniards? What about the South American Incans, or the Mayans? Ancient America had farm animals and large populations, up to millions of people living in interconnected clusters together, *empires*. The idea of civilisation-bred microbes doesn't settle this one: as if it's supposed to be obvious that llama and guinea pig microbes aren't as dangerous/powerful as cow and horse microbes (llama, turkey, alpaca and whatever other exclusively-American animals that were domesticated).

If we are going to invoke savage animal-originating microbes, are we going to assume horses and cows have more powerful microbes than the marsupials of Australia? No other humans had encountered most of those marsupials before the Australian Aboriginals. The Aboriginals lived close to these marsupials for probably over 50 thousand years, and they'd also lived with ungulate (hoofed) mammals in the past, so really, the Aboriginals would have had the edge in the microbe battle, against the Europeans who've *also* evolved alongside ungulated placental-mammal viruses but have seemingly never evolved alongside marsupial viruses. Theoretically, the Australian aboriginal population would have undergone unique selection pressures living with these microbes; it just takes one successful mutation to infect a human and kick off from there a major culling of the people, leaving the survivors with a microbial weapon against human lineages that haven't yet encountered the microbe. We hear no report of deadly Aussie, Kiwi, Solly or American microbes ravaging Europeans abroad or back home during the major European invasion days. We can only reasonably declare that community devastation increases the disease rates of those living in the community.

The Maori people of New Zealand were not notably ravaged by smallpox or measles, although they did endure a higher than usual disease rate during their standoff with the Europeans—their whole culture had been significantly disrupted, their nutriment sources and patterns, and their beneficial and essential communal processions were significantly affected—but in total, the NZ European invasion seems to be the least harsh out of American NZ and Australian invasions. There was no reason why the Maori people were not to be ravaged by smallpox and measles if it's all about immunology. Some people are even disinclined to call the European occupation of NZ an invasion.

In 1891, Maori member of parliament James Carrol reportedly said, "I am forced to the conclusion that it is a mistaken theory that the native race will rapidly decrease" (Raeburn Lange, 'Te hauora Māori i mua – history of Māori health - Health devastated, 1769 to 1901', Te Ara - the Encyclopedia of New Zealand). I think he is right—it's not a rule of thumb. Imagine if the Europeans arrived as slaves to the aboriginals, and the aboriginals bullied them and had the guns whilst the Europeans had no metal: reverse the roles. If the aboriginals fed their European prisoners food their lineage had never eaten before (probably also mostly undesirable or rotten), raped, bashed and murdered some of the Europeans regularly, hung dead European children around the European 'enclosures', I'm sure it would appear to some contagion-believers as though the aboriginals must-have given the Europeans a plague, as the Europeans get sick and *wither away in a similar manner*: because aboriginal people are fine eating that food and *they shouldn't be too stressed-out that it would affect their physiology drastically*, apparently. When Carrol said this in 1891, the Maori population was increasing.

The biggest account of smallpox in New Zealand was in 1913—which was 260-plus years after the first recorded

European contact—55 people died
(https://teara.govt.nz/en/epidemics/page-4). There must have
been more people vaccinated against smallpox at this time, in
this country, than ever before. This epidemic occurred six
years after Great Britain decided mandatory vaccination was
not justified (reference: the first chapter of this book).

There were many species of large flightless bird—*ratites*, the
same kind of bird as the Australian emus and cassowaries,
and the ostrich (called "moa")—that the Maori people ate and
would have acquired new, unique microbes from directly—
and, as a result of their altered body chemistry, cultivated new
microbe strains. *This could have helped them during the
invasion.* The NZ Kiwi bird is a ratite but not a Moa "There
ain't no Moa in old Aotearoa. Cant get 'em. They've et 'em; They've
gone and there ain't no Moa" – I am not sure who the originator
of these song lyrics is. Moa's and Kiwi birds, both being
ratites, are more closely related to birds that have been found
on other continents. The. Maori's ate to extinction about 9
different species of Moa, all flightless and large.

It seems (in the universities) that the Maori people were only
in New Zealand for perhaps 700 years before the Europeans
got there, but in that time, they managed to have a war
whereby at one time 10,000 people were actively involved
(the Battle of Hingakaka, apparently started from *accusations
of poorly distributed fish stock*). A group of people arrived in
canoes—I'd say 35 people—finding an amazing abundance
of nutriment, specifically *large flightless birds*, and several
hundred years later, 10,000 of their descendants became
actively involved in warfare against each other. When
European technology arrived, mayhem erupted, and the
Maoris formed a kind of small integrated island empire of their
own, fought against the Europeans with European tech, and
made a name for themselves and secured a decent deal with
the unstopping Europeans. They also went to the Chatham
Islands with this tech and committed genocide; notably, the
Chatham Island people were said to be of the same lineage
that originally arrived in NZ. Many people who consider

themselves *Kiwi* have taken to believing that a race of people had occupied New Zealand *before* the Maori, namely the Mori Ori. This seems to be a misconception that the Kiwi people have taken up from twisted facts: "The Mori Ori were in New Zealand first" = apparent fact ... "The Maori Killed all of the Mori Ori" = apparent fact ...

Somehow, a rift has started whereby people are adamantly telling me, an Australian, that the Maori weren't the first to populate New Zealand and that they killed and ate the native humans, *who had fuzzy red hair*. Again, the Mori Ori *were* exterminated by the Maori, and the Mori Ori *were* the first people in New Zealand. The twist forms because they were the same people as the Maori who first arrived at New Zealand, who further migrated away from New Zealand to Chatham Islands and became a distinct culture. My mother's mother was more Maori than she was not.

One last seemingly random piece of information about New Zealand: A giant eagle, weighing some 13 kilograms and possessing a wingspan of three metres, and was most definitely eating those big moa birds, has become extinct, most likely because the Maoris outhunted it rather than hunted it ... the biggest eagle to have flown on earth, as far as the universities can tell circa 2020.

Germm Theory

Germ theory seems to be the self-fulfilling prophecy of the original and primordial belief in Supernatural Origins of Harm, of finding strain-specific disease-associated microbes. All along, as far as history is recorded and even after finding microbes with microscopes, we have believed that disease comes in the form of a curse or conquest upon one's self. The revolution and progression in ideology—to me—seems to be the cessation of idealising that one is ever under attack or conquest by some intangible agent or force.

If germ theory is an accurate account of reality, then wearing a two-way-filtered mask is working to hold-in any viruses that are born in your lungs, where they have a chance to infect more respiratory cells. It seems to me that, according to the mainstream theory of disease genesis 2020, wearing a mask would provide an obstacle to the newborn microbes that would otherwise be *exhaled rather than propagated...* perhaps this is why I can't find one controlled experiment where mask-wearing coincided with *an actual lowering* of disease incidence or infectious-disease diagnoses, although my best bet is that germ-theory/contagion is an inaccurate depiction of reality and this is why the experimental findings don't support the dominant belief circa 2020.

The German-born PhD virologist and molecular biologist Stefan Lanka has done a lot of work in this area of science (disease genesis). He is not the only PhD biologist to disbelieve in contagious diseases in 2020, but he is the most famous one of them alive, surely due to his work in the German courthouses. Lanka won a case against a medical doctor in the German Supreme Court over precisely what is known (scientific evidence) about the measles virus ... he won

84

the case after losing in the lower court. Lanka would have had to have given out 100 thousand euros if someone met his challenge criteria, which the medical doctor David Bardens was convinced he had done (it was a challenge regarding scientific evidence, issued by Stefan), yet the supreme court judge ruled in Lanka's favour. If you Google searched this story in 2020, you are likely to have only found the propaganda that was put out almost immediately when the lower court ruled that David Bardens had sufficed the challenge criteria. For whatever reason, the much meatier story whereby the highest courthouse in the country ruled that the challenge criteria had not been met, didn't get the same kind of media launch and residue.

The exposé that viruses aren't self-replicating organisms is Lanka's most distinguished work. Lanka has seemingly revealed the human craftsmanship in working micro particles into a theory of a self-replicating package of genetically-arranged material which reproduces itself via catalysing X-cells to take it in and produce more copies of it, rather than these observed particles being unfolded, extricated, secreted or excreted components of X-cells.

That this has possibly happened, that we have potentially cooked up this big theory of viruses which is far from reality, begs the question why/how? It seems that the pre-existing and ancient conviction that characters of disease were *acquired*, and the finding of disease-specific particles/material, led to the development of this theory: To find/declare a material culprit for disease characters that occur in synchronicity within human populations and within plants like tobacco mosaic virus, was demanded by a culture that already believed disease was coming from outside as a kind of conquest upon the affected organism. Many 'viruses' were discovered and declared before they were able to be seen, like the first virus ever declared to have been found (tobacco mosaic virus), and like the human polio virus and more. This virus theory fit the pre-existing ideological paradigm, as most people would have already believed it was in fact a truth that *at least some* characters of disease were acquired from *a conquering agent*. And there's another reason, perhaps the most significant one:

'Virus' particle/material, when experimented-with under the belief that it is the cause of disease-transference, did just as much as bacteria and fungus with regard to causing/transferring disease. We had observed fungus and bacteria to be self-replicating organisms, and we had blamed them for causing the diseases they were associated-with. In terms of causing cellular-destruction and/or "disease" in experiments: virus, fungus and bacteria all appear to have the same kind of effective profile: in controlled experiments inconsistent with the measured nature/reality of microbial-contact (frequency and concentration), a cause of disease has been pronounced using all three—virus, bacteria and fungus. We seemingly *cannot* pronounce disease by introducing a theoretically disease-causing microbe to its theoretically–disease-caused organism when keeping consistent with the *frequency* and *concentration* of microbe-to-host contact.

Lanka has seemingly uncovered a delusion—one that was born from the self-fulfilling prophecy of our ancient belief in disease-contagion, and the findings and chemical analyses of disease-specific bio-particles/material associated with communally synchronised disease characters (like measles). Lanka is currently working to influence a better understanding of appropriate control forms in virological experimentation. Here is a link to one prominent article of his, from a website where you can find a lot more about his work and more: https://wissenschafftplus.de/uploads/article/Dismantling-the-Virus-Theory.pdf

This is a YouTube link to a video I made encapsulating what I've found to be the most prominent points on this matter (including key outcomes of Dr Lanka's experiments): I believe Dr Lanka has produced—in a laboratory—materials which read as COVID19 under PCR-detection (according to common/standard diagnostic guidelines for PCR etc), without the addition of any COVID19 sample, just using pathogen-free human cells and conditional arrangements/divisions: https://youtu.be/f49UYesrrC0. The contended delusion of contagious diseases is the overarching one; to me, it appears as the rotten root that has wrought the hollow branch of virology (recently exposed by Lanka) as well as the useless and dangerous fruit *vaccination*.

Imagine...

Imagine we could shrink ourselves as much as we like. And imagine we are farming epithelial cells, feeding them, nurturing them ... The germ-theorist farmer is worried about microbial predators, whereas Lanka is only concerned about the health of the epithelial cells. Again and again I have said in this book and will say (hopefully in *nuanced* ways): as far as I'm aware, no microbe has proven to be dangerous to any organism in controlled experimental conditions featuring the introduction of the microbe in quantities that are consistent with the given microbe's prevalence within environments that are naturally hosting the organism and contaminated with the microbe, featuring disease associated with that microbe for the organism. What I'm saying is, no one appears to have replicated a natural disease transmission in circumstances consistent with reality. For example, Bd fungus is said to be the primary cause of the extinction of many frog species since 1970. How prevalent is the Bd fungus in the natural environment? how many zoospores per millilitre of water are in naturally contaminated ponds, and how frequent are the frogs in them / how did a mass-extinction start allegedly from introducing a few spores to an environment? We should be able to imitate realistic conditions of theoretical infection and produce it in controlled experiments; we should be able to simply grow this fungus upon frog cells as the frog is destroyed, yet this does not appear to have been achieved throughout our endeavours to do so. Somehow, we as a culture in 2020 have afforded the best guess that the marching extinction of frog species since the 70s is due to poor quarantine measures, as different strains of the Bd fungus were introduced from abroad all over the world.

I am catering for the fact that these undertaking microbes *might* be a necessary part of the upkeep of complex organisms such as ourselves. As we all know, a house should be renovated often to suit the changing times so that the host can function most viably. Some people seem to have work being done on/to their house the whole time they are living in it, some people never complete every job in their house and they get by like this, without the luxury of a fully functioning house or workshop (like many Bd-infected frogs on earth currently, spending their whole lives enduring a light load of disease). Refurbishing needs to happen; sometimes whole walls, roofs, doors or plumbing systems need replacing because sometimes things fall out of place and need deconstructing and reconstructing (sometimes perfectly fine parts of the house need to be demolished along with broken parts in order to fix the overall problem). Sometimes parts/functions of the facility need to be disabled or retarded in-order-to / whilst-we refurbish others. We cannot function well in a house with mouldy walls, clogged plumbing and a leaking roof, or in a house that simply isn't designed well for what the host wants/needs. We need to refurbish these cellular structures and renovate to keep up with the changing times, and the manner in which this fixing mechanism has manifested appears to often be associated with microbial interaction (maintenance agents), also involving the cellular degeneration-into, and perhaps even ingestion-of, materials we are at this stage calling "virus".

The reason food doesn't rot quicker in the fridge isn't because bacteria are slower when it's cold—it's because the enzymes within the food in the fridge are working slower. Bacteria and fungus feed on spoilt food; the micro eruptions of the enzymic activity that are constantly occurring form the changing terrain that initiates microbial proliferation... Abrupt climate change doesn't make the beetle more savage: it provides more degenerated/beetle-available tree structures for the beetles than usual, which results in more beetle activity (I'm talking to *you, Martin J Blaser* (reference the Rocky Mountains pine forest degeneration issue, mentioned in Martin's book 'Missing Microbes')).

The reason anti-microbial wound-dressing suddenly seemed appropriate around the end of the 1800s was because Joseph Lister experimented and found that it has the general effect of increasing healing speed. The whole antibiotics usage and impression (especially during WW2) is an extrapolation of this original observation which, *tied together with germ theory and vaccination*, has managed to absolutely dominate as an ideological force: civilian: "my son/husband healed because of the medication"; physician: "this medication speeds the process up (decision/determination), and thus keeps the hospitals freer": it seems well settled that no one has ever proven in controlled experiments that antimicrobial wound dressing or the ingestion of antibiotics will increase the overall chances of healing, only a hastening thereof. Increasing the healing speed through intervention effected the illusion to common human observers that "the chances of healing at all" have increased as a result of the intervention.

Frog Apocalypse

I believe this case study, featuring the fungus *Batrachochytrium dendrobatidis* (AKA 'Bd'), is very important and relative to our culture's understanding and approach to disease-science. Some frogs are found to be healthy whilst this fungus is growing with/in/on them, although the fungus appears to be associated with a lot of the amphibian deaths occurring: this is popularly hypothesised to be due to the disease-causing nature of the particular fungus, and the virulence of specific Bd strains to specific frog species.

Since sequencing the genome of Bd fungus, we have found it to be on every major continent except for Antarctica. The most popular explanation for why so many frogs are dying with this fungus growing in/on/with them, in otherwise pristine environments, is *poor quarantine measures*: Bd spores have been introduced by us, infesting frog species that haven't seen them before and rendering them extinct.

The less popular theory suggests that since we have devastated many environmental niches, we have abruptly changed the chemical profile of the worldwide environment, which has caused problems for the inhabitants of this environment, frogs being a primary or 'indicative' concern. With all our activity, which includes—amongst other factors—environmental pollution and deforestation, these otherwise pristine environments with sudden amphibian-disease epidemics aren't actually pristine, they are disrupted and damaged on an unseen and thus-far-unmeasured level. Us humans only notice the frogs dying, without a definitive trace, and we blame the fungus in accordance with how we as a culture think about microbial-associated disease genesis.

Many people are suggesting a mix of these two theories: that we have devastated the environment, the frogs have become susceptible and we have introduced a deadly fungus which is able to devastate the susceptible frog populations. In 1998, after considering the apparent frog population demise, we set out to understand what was going on, and we sequenced the genome of a fungus that was frequenting most of these diseased frogs to a measurable degree. Scientists identified a "chytrid" fungus called Batrachochytrium dendrobatidis (Bd), and we are now finding variants all over the world.

A frog that was preserved in South Africa in 1938 has been found to have *the fungus* in it, and originally this was the earliest one known. We have recently found a frog preserved in Japan from 1908 in which the Bd signature was positively detected. Another account I saw from the NCBI website said, 'Bd has been present in the USA for at least 140 years, with the oldest records from southern leopard frogs (Lithobates sphenocephala) collected in Illinois in 1888' (Lips KR. Overview of chytrid emergence and impacts on amphibians. Philos Trans R Soc Lond B Biol Sci. 2016;371(1709):20150465. doi:10.1098/rstb.2015.0465 https://www.ncbi.nlm.nih.gov/pmc/articles/PMC5095542/). I'm wondering how deep we have searched through the frog records in the museums (what the oldest sample we can test is).

Currently, it is being popularly hypothesised that the fungus originated in Korea ('A plague from South Korea is killing frogs and toads worldwide' https://www.newscientist.com/article/2168568-a-plague-from-south-korea-is-killing-frogs-and-toads-worldwide/). The strongest evidence supporting the sole blame of the spread of Bd spores as the cause of all these frogs that have died and the species that have become extinct, seems to be *the measured 'marching spread'* of the Bd associated disease in "otherwise pristine environments". As we see a spreading disease epidemic only in frogs, we assume the fungus is the primary issue with the environment. Here is a reported observation in central America of a north to south spread, and other marching/progressing spreads around the region: (Lips KR, Brem F, Brenes R, Reeve JD, Alford RA, Voyles J, Carey C, Livo L, Pessier AP, Collins JP, 2006. Emerging infectious disease and the loss of biodiversity in a Neotropical amphibian community. Proceedings of the National Academy of Sciences of the United States of America, 103(9):3165-3170. http://www.pnas.org/). The idea that the marching spread is caused by the spread of the fungus is easy to understand, although it's not easily understood nor commonly agreed upon why the experiments we have conducted thus far don't support this idea very well, *if at all* ...

The marching spread of a microbial-level ecological breakdown is understandable, and it seems reasonable to suggest that a significant change in the chemical procession/profile of the environment would characterise this change, and the only thing us humans would notice is the first line of species to become heavily diseased and perhaps subsequently extinct ... It seems reasonable to suggest that the world environment has received abrupt increases of "pollution" in terms of effect from the material combinations within earth's pre-existing ecosystem, both from our rubbish and our destruction of pre-existing ecosystems (systems which are connected beyond rainforest boundaries). It seems the only other time such a red-blooded animal extinction has taken place was when a meteorite larger than 9km in diameter collided with the earth, triggering major ecosystem disruptions and *ipso facto extinctions*. It seems reasonable to suggest we currently are in a similar situation in terms of pollution (stability of ecosystem, in terms of the rate at which red-blooded animals go extinct and come to development/distinction). It seems reasonable to say the ecosystem will collapse on an unseen (to the human eye) level first, and that this collapse will move in a marching direction (a marching chemical alteration, like "pasture dieback" in grasslands). The experimental findings we have accrued thus far seem to be most compatible with my alternative hypothesis.

Frogs are known to be an indicator species, meaning when something happens to them, it signifies a significant change in the ecosystem has taken place. The demise of the frogs themselves would initiate major changes in the ecosystem, but the preceding changes may be unnoticed to us: microbial-level ecological collapse and micro-ecological dieback, causing a major change (extraordinary) in environmental chemistry wherever the collapse has been effected, and spreading outwards from wherever the collapse has occurred *in a marching fashion*.

What might cause the marching microbial ecological collapse? Perhaps a myriad of things, most likely stemming from the activity of humans (perhaps human-induced climate change is involved; *most definitely pollution and environmental destruction*). Other species of fungus have been noted for having incredibly large networks, so when one area of an environment is poisoned or impoverished, it may affect another area many miles away, through the mycelium network, and in other ways like groundwater. Oceans, rivers and the air, are like highways for ecosystems, connecting them together.

Imagine the whole biosphere of a major rainforest area, including all the microbes, and the chemistry *that* is, constantly working out a process that has settled in over millions of years (for however long the rainforest has existed!) ... Imagine that setting being abruptly polluted (with or without climate change), and a cessation of the rainforest's primordial microbial activity patterns occurs—mayhem would erupt, chemically speaking: this would be a disaster for the organisms in that rainforest which have evolved a certain chemistry that functions optimally for the ancient rainforest ecosystem/pattern. Humans wouldn't know anything was amiss until the frogs started dying. It seems to me likely that the chemical cycle *falls out* in one spot first and spreads like fire from there, like a marching chemical fallout/storm, summed up as "mostly-human–caused environmental devastation/pollution".

Amphibiosis. For all we know, Bd fungus is an amphibiotic microbe: a certain path of disease may ensue with Bd as the frogs' only chance of survival in the abruptly-changed chemical circumstances. I mean, for all we know at this stage—and I'd bet this is the case—Bd fungus flourishing on/in frogs is the subsequent result of cellular-incapacity (cellular-chemistry failure). Perhaps the fungus strain has been evolving with amphibians all along, as a necessary part of the organism, and the recent abrupt chemical changes have triggered the relationship to become more tense as the frogs are environmentally stressed and require extraordinary chemical-alteration within themselves (disease) in order to survive. Perhaps the fungus has been carried through the amphibian lineages, passed over through offspring, evolving over many generations with the animal, lying dormant and playing a certain role in/as the biology of the amphibians. Some Bd strains may have only recently arisen with the recent *major changes* on earth—*chemically speaking*. These environments, before breaking down into frog disease epidemics, may reach a kind of boiling point, a crescendo where once reached, things start falling drastically out of place (chemically speaking).

I find it hard to conceive that we have any pristine environments left, given the earth's atmosphere is one shared environment and it has been abruptly altered, including the ocean, which affects the inland environment through chain effects. Any pristine environment that appears fine to us may be disturbed from a chain reaction of a disrupted ecology some 500 kilometres away (or perhaps even anywhere on earth) that has marched to this otherwise pristine environment on a microbial level, eventuating through the butterfly effect and disrupting the otherwise-pristine environment without a trace.

'Molecular evidence appears to suggest that the global spread of Bd was a recent event'

(Morehouse EA, James TY, Ganley ARD, Vilgalys R, Berger L, Murphy PJ, Longcore JE, 2003. Multilocus sequence typing suggests the chytrid pathogen of amphibians is a recently emerged clone. Molecular Ecology, 12(2):395-403

James TY, Litvintseva AP, Vilgalys R, Morgan JAT, Taylor JW, Fisher MC, Berger L, Weldon C, Preez L du, Longcore, JE, 2009. Rapid Global Expansion of the Fungal Disease Chytridiomycosis into Declining and Healthy Amphibian Populations. PLoS Pathogens, 5(5):e1000458).

A famous PhD biologist, Rupert Sheldrake, has reported that we have evidence of a certain crystal structure that wasn't recorded before, which all of a sudden manifested in one lab, and then another lab, and another, all over the world. He claims there seems to be some kind of crystal intelligence that permeates throughout existence. I wonder if this might be happening with other things, such as fungus ... or else birds have transported new strains around the world. Or, perhaps, some are airborne and can travel in clouds, like other known fungal spores. Although I'd bet Bd can't travel in clouds, maybe some strains of the spores *can*, just like some other fungus species. Sheldrake brought in the 'morphic resonance' theory/book, suggesting this kind of intelligence is shared amongst all organisms. I am in no way leaning on this theory to support my own regarding the spread of Bd-associated disease in frogs—hence I haven't included any links or references to his studies/work (I'm just sharing this much from what I've read over time). The recent spread of many of these strains of Bd is likely to be associated with the recent drastic changes in the worldwide environment: significantly new terrain equals significantly new strains. I'd bet that Bd fungus is as old as amphibians themselves.

I typed "infecting frogs with BD experiment" into Google to find out about some experiments that sought to prove the mechanism of this fungus' acquisition and pathogenicity, and the first one I found was very interesting (Byrne AQ, Poorten TJ, Voyles J, Willis CKR, Rosenblum EB. Opening the file drawer: Unexpected insights from a chytrid infection experiment. *PLoS One*. 2018;13(5):e0196851. Published 2018 May 9. doi:10.1371/journal.pone.0196851, https://www.ncbi.nlm.nih.gov/pmc/articles/PMC5942794/?fbclid=I

wAROznXcTUYOyveyhwgnKXWDgvwL-
e9cyFl0QI4DUtkyvwiR2aKAntvVptqU). This experiment turns out to be very significant to me, because it highlights some interesting and pertinent facts: frogs can be Bd-negative, and become Bd-positive in controlled conditions (experimental). The infecting Bd strain found on the uninoculated frog was a strain that wasn't introduced to any of the frogs in the experiment—this frog was *a control frog* which is used to help us see if the Bd being introduced to frogs in the experiment can harm the frogs: the control frogs are there to control for the confounding factor of frogs being put through extraordinary conditions which could themselves harm them. The Bd in this frog is likely to have been within the frog when it was screened with the PCR test, and evaded detection (perhaps just spores).

In other words, some frogs were *mock-inoculated* yet became detectably-infected with Bd fungus during the trial. This indicates that Bd spores can remain dormant and undetected because the frog was in a controlled environment and had previously passed negative for Bd right before being placed into the controlled environment—this is accounted-for by the authors and most–if-not-all microbiologists.

In this most-recently mentioned experiment, two species of frog: one (*R. Muscosa*) considered highly susceptible to the particular Bd being used, another (*R. catesbeiana)* which is considered not so susceptible to the Bd. Both frog species were inoculated with the Bd, and both species constituted a "control" group which received everything included in the inoculation process (a bath in certain solution, etc.) minus the Bd spores: this is what we call a *sham inoculation*, used to clear up any chance of disease occurring from the inoculation process itself irrespective of Bd. In my opinion, such sham inoculations should include spores from another species of fungus that isn't associated with disease in the animal to control the potentially compromising factor of having electro-chemical packages present in the bath water, and obviously the control zoospores should be of a similar biomass/quantity, *action* and chemistry to the experimental challenge ones (all microbial challenge experiments should have this control, and yet I've never seen it: similar biomass of a similar species or strain of microbe that isn't associated with disease in the given organism).

> Bd-inoculated *R. catesbeiana* (n = 20), sham-inoculated *R. catesbeiana* (n = 20), Bd-inoculated *R. muscosa* (n = 18), and sham-inoculated *R. muscosa* (n = 19).

Interestingly, as I've already gone-over, some uninoculated frogs (*R. catesbeiana*) became Bd positive *during* the experiment with a strain that wasn't used in the experiment, *perhaps because the experimental settings disrupted the chemical balance of the frogs and a dormant Bd strain manifested to a measurable degree as it thus had some work to do (chemical balancing).* This indicates that any other experiment, where some frogs became Bd positive, may have been due to the stress the experimental setting inflicted upon the frog (which is characterised by chemical change), causing subsequent Bd manifestation and antibody production. For all we know, this may be the most reasonable physiological path for the frog that chemically falls out of balance. In experiments where frogs become Bd-positive and diseased (rare apparently, although I'll share what I've found of this sort) after being inoculated with Bd, we should test to see if the strain they became positive with is the same as the one they were inoculated with: 'We found that the *R. catesbeiana* control frogs were not infected with the Bd isolate that we used for inoculations (CJB5-2), but rather a significantly diverged Bd isolate'—alas, from this experiment, it is written: 'In the Bd-inoculated *R. catesbeiana* treatment group, the inoculated genotype appeared to out-compete the cryptic infection.' it was confirmed—*not just from that sentence*—that the Bd used in the experiment did occupy to a measurable degree the inoculated frogs. I don't know enough about PCR to comment here on how certain anyone can be about the relations of infecting Bd fungus strains according to PCR readings, but I have learnt all I sense needs to be learnt to assess the performance dynamics of vaccination and microbes.

These frogs were inoculated with 1 x 10^6 (1 million) zoospores, in 30ml of liquid (20% Holtfretter's solution), for 24 hours, and the control frogs had the same bath except without the zoospores (which, electro-chemically speaking, to me, is a significantly different bath for a frog). The frogs were then monitored for 10 weeks, some had Bd infections develop (including uninoculated frogs) detected by PCR. Zoospores move around, hence the prefix *zoo*, stemming from *animal* (locomotives).

During this trial, three of the control frogs died "for unknown reasons" (the considered highly susceptible *R. Muscosa*), and one of the experimental frogs died from a broken leg (subsequently euthanised):

> We hypothesized that *R. catesbeiana* would be more resistant to Bd infection, show lower Bd loads, less negative change in body mass, less mortality, and more antibody-mediated immunity than *R.muscosa*. However, we were surprised to find no mortality in the highly-susceptible *R. muscosa* and no evidence of antibody-mediated immunity in either species. Moreover, during the experiment one of our control groups became unexpectedly Bd-positive. Our study was initially relegated to the file drawer because of these anomalous results, but after developing a new Bd genotyping assay, we were able to diagnose the source of one important anomaly and gain new insights into disease dynamics in this system.

> In fact, we observed no Bd-related mortality in any of our treatment groups. All *R. muscosa* Bd-exposed individuals survived for the duration of the experiment, although three *R. muscosa* in the control group died during week 6 for unknown reasons. All R. catesbeiana individuals in the control group survived the duration of the experiment, while one individual in the *R. catesbeiana* Bd-exposed group was euthanized during week 6 because of a broken leg.

It seems there was no problem with contacting Bd for any of the frogs in this experiment, although it did come into detection with some of them (not sure if they were the challenge strains of Bd that were measured or some other strain, but they were Bd). Maybe the highly susceptible R Mucosa frogs that featured in this study benefitted from the Bd that was introduced to them, and the dead ones missed out... Frogs are likely disturbed by chemical profile changes in their environment, falling into disease when it affects their own balance of chemistry; just because we find Bd involved in the terrible situation of cellular failure doesn't mean the situation would be better without Bd, or that Bd-acquisition *caused* the situation. Again, the motorcycle moves predominantly because the gaseous material ignites and energy is released, not because *a sprocket turns a chain...*

> The Bd on swabs collected from *R. catesbeiana* and *R. muscosa* Bd-exposed frogs was positioned as expected in the phylogeny—forming a well-supported cluster with the inoculation isolate (CJB5-2, Fig 3). However, the mystery isolate was found in a distinct subclade within the Bd-GPL clade (Global Panzootic Lineage [42], Fig 3).

The above statement also confirms that the same Bd strain used in the experiment was detected to be occupying the frogs that were exposed to it.

Amphibiosis?

"But Bd is a pathogenic parasite, therefore this can't be a case of amphibiosis" (The Voice of The Culture). Things change, like what happened with the bacterium *H. pylori*—it was parasitic and pathogenic and now one of the head honchos (Martin Blaser) of western biomedicine is saying it's amphibiotic.

"I just really can't see how you can downplay the extreme virulence of Bd" (- The Voice of The Culture) = Because the first experiment that popped up on Google reported no problem for the Bd-inoculated highly-susceptible *R. muscosa* (yet three without the Bd died *for unknown reasons*), and a separate Bd strain manifested in some of the commonly unsusceptible frog species that weren't inoculated with the experimental strain of Bd. This caters for the hypothesis that Bd infections are environmentally induced and Bd is not disease-causing but rather disease-accompanying.

Surely it's more likely that the abrupt extinction of many frog species in the last 50 years is the result of humanity's pollution and destruction, rather than the spread of a fungus (which could theoretically spread at any moment to wipe out every animal, given the pathways are there for it, through birds, clouds, wind, and even the ocean).

<u>The Bd-load directly correlates with disease intensity during chytridiomycosis</u>. The heavier the cellular work is, the more Bd will be needed. We have found the disease-associated fungus and are inclined to blame it rather than blame our human activity, which is still continuing in such a destructive and pollutive manner.

More from this experiment report:

> Although infection experiments have tremendous value for understanding disease processes, there are potential pitfalls to experimental approaches. Disease outcomes are influenced by interactions among host, pathogen and environment [2]. The complexity of these interactions can affect the repeatability of infection experiments among laboratories or even within the same laboratory over time. This, in turn, can lead to ambiguous experimental results that are difficult to interpret, apply to disease management and conservation, and publish.

> The "file drawer" problem—where non-significant or ambiguous results are less likely to be published in the scientific literature [10]—is a longstanding issue in biological research. Not only are journals often biased against non-significant results [11,12], but researchers may be less likely to submit results that are inconsistent with past work and/or difficult to interpret [13]. The file drawer problem in wildlife disease research is a potentially significant obstacle to progress.

The way we are telling the story in the mainstream narrative, you would expect that we are able to simply place a specific zoospore or three on a specific frog and demonstrate disease genesis … just like how we may reasonably expect that we have demonstrated that we can spray a dog with a million parvo viruses and demonstrate disease genesis, or spray some flu viruses in the air for some brave participants to breathe in and demonstrate the mechanism of disease genesis. But we can't do anything of the sort. We can aerosolise materials containing a virus, and cause disease in organisms that way, but this involves a more extraordinary exposure method than that which occurs in reality (PPM and duration).

I eventually found some experiments that indicated microbe-introduction caused disease without any bodily injections in frogs, using BD spores, and you can decide if you think this is consistent with real-world circumstances. A friend, who is a zoologist, seemed angry at me for not just believing that Bd is the primary cause of the disease it features in; he seemed angry when I said I can't find any experiment that shows this … at me … with the full weight of all those recently-extinct amphibian species.

(Frog microbiome disturbance by a fungal pathogen Andrea J. Jani, Cheryl J. Briggs Proceedings of the National Academy of Sciences Nov 2014, 111 (47) E5049-E5058; DOI:10.1073/pnas.1412752111 https://www.pnas.org/content/111/47/E5049). After looking harder for proof that some frogs have been killed with Bd in experiments, I found a study that indicates a disparity between what we think is the reality and what actually is, *although*: 'Despite these differences in disease dynamics, the relationship between BD load and bacterial community composition was documented across all four populations'.

This report hypothesises that BD affects the bacterial microbiome of the frogs and *that's* linked to causing the disease. Basically, the experiment was set to prove the pathogenic nature of Bd, and the outcomes weren't so straightforward, but some interesting findings were established, like the bacterial ecology alteration within the microbiome of the frogs after being inoculated with Bd. Add a load of X chemical package to the mucous layer of a frog's skin, and you will likely change the bacterial demographic.

Another article on Bd from the *Science* magazine reads as if it is established that we are justified in primarily blaming poor quarantine measures and Bd for killing frogs and other amphibians. (Pathogenesis of Chytridiomycosis, a Cause of Catastrophic Amphibian Declines Science 23 Oct 2009: Vol. 326, Issue 5952, pp. 582-585 DOI: 10.1126/science.1176765) The most interesting part, to me, was this: "The pathogenesis of chytridiomycosis has been difficult to determine because cutaneous fungal infections are rarely fatal without other predisposing factors", a statement which comes with the reference to "M. Schaechter, B. I. Eisensteing, G. Medoff, in *Mechanisms of Microbial Disease* (Williams & Wilkins, Baltimore, 1998), pp. 419–439". In other words, simply putting Bd on the skin of the frog doesn't kick-off disease, yet we afford ourselves the mainstream narrative that most of these frog species that have gone-extinct in the last 50 years did-so due-to poor quarantine-measures.

Another article (Distribution of the amphibian chytrid Batrachochytrium dendrobatidis and keratin during tadpole development GERRY MARANTELLP, LEE BERGER2,3*, RICK SPEARE2 and LEIGH KEEGAW https://www.researchgate.net/profile/Lee_Berger2/publication/279 595290_Distribution_of_the_amphibian_chytrid_Batrachochytrium _dendrobatidis_and_keratin_during_tadpole_development/links/55 9cfcbb08ae4e46ea2074ae/Distribution-of-the-amphibian-chytrid-Batrachochytrium-dendrobatidis-and-keratin-during-tadpole-development.pdf), from the early days of Bd detection reports that a whole heap of tadpoles had survived up until they metamorphosed into frogs. The tadpoles were found to have Bd growing on their mouths, *which is the only keratinised part of the tadpole* (able to support Bd occupation). When the frogs develop from the tadpole, and the skin begins to develop, this is when the fungus occupies a significant amount of the frog, as it occupies the skin of the frog. Perhaps these tadpoles came from a line of unhealthy frogs from an unhealthy ecosystem and the poor health carried over to the offspring. Health/vitality seems to be like a bank in that it can be built up for an organism: the healthier an organism, the more proficient it will be at building reproductive cells, and this health/vitality can be built up and also broken down over generations. In this case study, when the tadpole stage is over, these tadpoles aren't constituted well enough to grow into frogs, and it's insinuated that the only issue with the tadpoles was they had Bd on their lips, which wouldn't allow them to grow their frog skin ... It seems an unhealthy population of frogs (probably just on the edge of demise) produced tadpoles that were placed in conditions outside of their natural environment for human observation, and the tadpoles didn't have it in them to grow as frogs in and after the experimental environment that they were put in.

> Infection of embryonic stages appears unlikely as they lack keratinized surfaces, but the potential of *B. dendrobatidis* to infect egg capsules needs to be investigated by experimental infection.

> Ecological studies are needed to determine the impact of chytridiomycosis on population structures.

The first experimental study article I found that *suggests* BD causes morbidity (Proc. Natl. Acad. Sci. USA Vol. 95, pp. 9031–9036, July 1998 Population Biology Chytridiomycosis causes amphibian mortality associated with population declines in the rain forests of Australia and Central America LEE BERGERa,b,c, RICK SPEAREa, PETER DASZAKd, D. EARL GREENEe, ANDREW A. CUNNINGHAMf, C. LOUISE GOGGINg, RON SLOCOMBEh, MARK A. RAGANi, ALEX D. HYATTb, KEITH R. MCDONALDj, HARRY B. HINESk, KAREN R. LIPSl, GERRY MARANTELLlm, AND HELEN PARKESb) is a well-documented account of the history of Bd's genetic sequencing, anatomy, and the process of its featuring in cellular degradation: what it does and how. Also, some more accounts are provided of healthy tadpoles with Bd on their keratinised lips becoming diseased as/after they transformed into frogs with keratinised skin over their body. Address to study: https://www.jstor.org/stable/45880

This report also refers to the 'seemingly pristine' environments. To rule out my alternative hypothesis, we need to measure the precise microbial ecology (inside and outside of the multicellular structures) of these environments before and after the disease epidemic. We can do this in areas where there is little to no amphibian decimation (I think some still exist), but this would constitute a vast amount of work, and would need major sponsoring, which would be hard in a world that is tranced in blaming the featuring agents of disease processes (seemingly mistaking consequence for cause).

As for the experiment:

> 14 frogs (6 exposed, 8 controls) from the previously sampled cohort were used. Each of six frogs was exposed to 800 ml of an aqueous suspension of approximately 3×10^3 sporangia in fresh skin scrapings taken from a dead frog of the same species that had naturally acquired cutaneous chytridiomycosis. Four frogs were exposed to water that had contained infected skin scrapings and had been passed through a 0.45-$\Box$m filter, and four were kept as untreated controls.

I don't know how much of this diseased skin was included in these frogs' bath, or what the precise chemical constitution of it was, but it allegedly contained 3000 Bd spores. I have no idea what chemical packages were filtered out for the controlled frog bath, but I would bet the Bd spores weren't the bulk of it, because if the zoospores could be filtered out, much of the skin scrapings would have been too. *How long were they in the bath for (e.g. the whole time)?*

> Between 10 and 18 days postexperimental exposure, all six frogs exposed to unfiltered skin scrapings became moribund; one died and the rest were euthanized with 0.2% tricaine methanesulfonate (Ruth

Consolidated Industries, Annandale, Australia). Cutaneous chytridiomycosis was diagnosed cytologically, histologically, and ultrastructurally. The eight control frogs remained healthy and were free of chytrids when killed after 22 days and examined histologically.

Why euthanise the survivors? Perhaps they would have recovered. There is no mention of how long after their bath they were killed or if they even were allowed out of their filthy bath water. In the next trial that I analyse, we find the frogs were submerged in the bath throughout the entire duration of the experiment. We have seen in the previously mentioned trial that some frogs testing negative for Bd can subsequently become positive for Bd whilst held in controlled experimental conditions with no Bd inoculation. Perhaps the frogs that took a bath in the unfiltered diseased-skin scrapings (which included Bd) developed illness /were poisoned from this filthy bath itself (chemically overwhelmed), and the inoculated Bd happened to become active during their illness, thus producing the "diagnosis" after their euthanasia; perhaps they became ill in the bath and dormant undetected strains of Bd manifested rather than the experimental strains. The fact that the euthanised sick frogs had Bd growing/in-occupation in/on their skin doesn't mean Bd caused their disease. Imagine if you took a bath in the skin scrapings of someone who had a major skin-disease which featured a fungus and, in that bath, with all the diseased-skin scrapings and fungus, you became very sick and your skin was rotting away with occupying funguses attending the site … Would you think you became sick only because of the fungus that was in the bath, because some other people took a bath in the same water as you *after* it was microfiltered (.45micron) and didn't get sick? Now imagine you're a frog ... frogs are much more dermatologically sensitive than we are.

Although the transmission experiment was a preliminary trial that used unpurified material, it demonstrates that chytrids are associated with a transmissible fatal disease of anurans and supports our diagnostic findings that cutaneous chytridiomycosis was the cause of the mortality events in wild amphibians.

105

I'm pretty sure it doesn't demonstrate *all that*—the experimental settings don't allow for it—but it does demonstrate what we already knew at that point: Bd occupation is often associated with disease procession, and frogs can be killed in various ways.

> Furthermore, the failure to identify alternative causes of death after examination of the wild amphibians and their environment (refs. 13 and 30; K.R.L., unpublished data) supports our theory that cutaneous chytridiomycosis was the cause of the riparian amphibian population declines in the montane rain forests of Queensland and Panama.

The failure to identify the complex chemical nature of organisms and environmental change and compatibility, microbial-level ecological-collapse, evolutionarily-abrupt changes, and the failure to identify the precise preceding stages and dynamics of cellular chemistry followed by Bd occupation give support to the following statement:

> The chytrid may be an introduced pathogen spreading through naïve populations (7, 8), or it may be a widespread organism that has emerged as a pathogen to frogs because of either an increase in virulence or an increased host susceptibility caused by other factors, such as environmental changes or as yet undetected coinfections.

The authors seem to not even entertain my point of view, which is alarming: they can't seem to imagine that the chemical-coordination of the frog cells is perhaps the only issue here, the Bd fungus is a biproduct of that, a consequence... And why would the cells have trouble coordinating chemistry? Maybe because everything about an ecosystem is chemically driven and these rainforest ecosystems on earth have been drastically altered recently (polluted).

I finally found what I was looking for: an experimental outcome of the allegedly rare nature, which showed *the addition of Bd spores alone* contributed to death. It is noted by some germ theory deniers that no animal is made sick from a microbe in ordinary circumstances of disease genesis (air sprayed or externally-applied in quantities and frequencies not significantly different to natural environmental circumstances). Here, we have semi-ordinary circumstances, whereby frogs—animals noted for their heightened skin sensitivity—are put with Bd zoospores, and made sick, whereby they either died or were euthanised.

I personally would bet that the frogs died because they were stuck for 30 days and nights in direct contact with a solution that contained a concentration of a chemical package (live organisms), which is not only electro-chemically problematic for the frog skin (skin comprised of bacteria amongst other cells) but a physical issue of forcefulness too: these microscopic zoospores are literally aerobic. It appears as though we are not dealing with a dangerous seed that can grow upon a susceptible frog if it so happens to be introduced to it, as this much is not pronounced in this experiment. The first line of contact to the environment for a healthy frog seems to be a well-kempt layer of mucous and bacteria. These chemical packages (zoospores) the frogs were forced to contact through a liquid medium were replenished weekly.

In this experimental study (Differential Host Susceptibility to Batrachochytrium dendrobatidis, an Emerging Amphibian Pathogen C. L. SEARLE,*§ S. S. GERVASI,* J. HUA,# J. I. HAMMOND,# R. A. RELYEA,# D. H. OLSON,† AND A. R. BLAUSTEIN* *Department of Zoology, Oregon State University, Corvallis, OR 97331, U.S.A. #Department of Biological Sciences, University of Pittsburgh, Pittsburgh, PA 15260, U.S.A. †United States Department of Agriculture, Forest Service, Pacific Northwest Research Station, Corvallis, OR 97331, U.S.A. https://www.biology.pitt.edu/sites/default/files/facilities-images/Searle.pdf) frogs had 260,000 zoospores added to the water that they were immersed in throughout the whole 30 days of the experiment: for the first week it appears as though there was only 15ml of liquid containing these zoospores, which is a rate of 17,333/ml, and after the water was changed (weekly) it is written that 10ml of water was added: it seems to be explicit that for the first week of the 30 days, the bath/inoculation liquid contained 17,333 zoospores/ml, and the rest of the time it contained 10400 zoospores/ml.

> Animals could partially climb the walls of the Petri dish, but could not completely lift themselves off the bottom; thus, they were in constant contact with the water. We kept animals in these dishes for the duration of the experiment (30 days) and fed them twice a week.

It seems beyond reasonable doubt that the essential difference between the frogs with Bd in their bath and the other frogs without Bd was the cause of most of the frogs dying in this experiment. This experiment doesn't confirm if the Bd that was found active with the dead frogs was the same strain as the Bd spores in the experiment. Overwhelming the frogs with zoospore chemical packages may have harmed them (and the Bd that grew on the degenerate cells could have grown from pre-existing Bd spores within the frog). The frogs surely wouldn't have been able to live a full life trapped in such an enclosure, and seemingly would die sooner if they featured the lofty concentration of zoospores in the water: constantly turning out protective peptides etc keeping their mucous layer nice and healthy.

As I said earlier, to get to the bottom of this we could add other chemical packages to the control frogs, similar to the zoospores ... perhaps we could use zoospores from another strain of chytrid fungus—or some other kind of fungus—that is found to be not disease-associated with the given species of frog; this would level out the control more. To add a similar amount of biomass in the form of zoospores to the control group's bath—this may even be a point of my originality. "Exposure to Bd increased mortality across species by a factor of 3.63."

Some of the species of frog in this experiment fared better than others.

Frogs make all kinds of chemical packages that are associated with upkeep processes in the skin. Frogs make more "antimicrobial peptides" (AMPs) than any other skinned animal, or *metazoan*, for that matter. It appears as though more study is needed in this area as to how exactly this all works. Here's an excerpt from Frog Skin Innate Immune Defences: 'Frog Skin Innate Immune Defences: Sensing and Surviving Pathogens Joseph F. A. Varga, Maxwell P. Bui-Marinos and Barbara A. Katzenback* Department of Biology, University of Waterloo, Waterloo, ON, Canada' under the heading 'Chemical Barriers', and the subheading 'Antimicrobial Peptides':

It is evident that AMPs serve a significant role in the defence of frog skin against pathogens, however our understanding of the ability of frog AMPs to exert antimicrobial activity on frog pathogens is limited and knowledge surrounding their potential immunomodulatory activity in frogs is completely lacking. (https://www.frontiersin.org/articles/10.3389/fimmu.2018.03128/full)

I'm betting we are not dealing with a dangerous seed of sorts, which is what is postulated to be the case given the mainstream *best guess* as to "why the marching frog extinctions?" being "poor quarantine measures". I'm betting we are dealing with a destabilised ecosystem, which ties-in with the definition of "pollution", and that we have blamed an associated and necessary entity of a specific disease-process for the disease-process itself, hence we are unable to develop any disease upon any cellular structure from the introduction of a single seed, as is evident in the literature.

The first and last experiments I found in my Frog Apocalypse investigation

The first one, where none of them developed the Bd-associated disease, but some became infected with Bd, and at least one which wasn't inoculated with Bd even became infected with Bd (which was confirmed to be of a different strain to the Bd used in the inoculation procedure): these frogs in this experiment were inoculated with 1 x *10 to the power of six* zoospores (one million) in 30 millilitres of water (33,333 zoospores per 1 ml) for 24 hours, and the control frogs had the same bath except without the zoospores and had the only mortalities (one due to broken leg, three due to unknown causes). The frogs were monitored for 10 weeks.

The last experiment I found (of the allegedly rare nature, according to M. Schaechter, B. I. Eisensteing, G. Medoff, in Mechanisms of Microbial Disease (Williams & Wilkins, Baltimore, 1998), pp. 419–439) showed very clear distinctions between Bd-inoculated frogs and non–Bd-inoculated frogs: these frogs were immersed in 15/25 ml of liquid with some 260 thousand zoospores for 30 days (17,333/10,400 zoospores per 1 ml).

Basically, the frogs that died with/from Bd averaged over one-third of the *load* of zoospores (given they had a ¼ of the number of zoospores in 5/6th of the amount of water) for a duration that was 30 times longer (involving unavoidable contact with the zoospore solution the whole time), as compared with the frogs that didn't die from the straight cut Bd introduction. If such a concentration of zoospores as 10,400/ml actually does present in nature, I'm sure no frog will be in forced-contact with this body of water for any amount of time (let alone 30 days).

COVID19: The Flowering of a Delusion

How did it start? Bill Gates et al.—rich people with lofty ambitions of being altruistic, have set the world up ready to be saved in an unprecedented manner ... a kind of plague-watch system was developed to the point where it took up a story based in China with two key assumptions: that the materials we have called "virus" all along really are the cause of the cellular processes they are associated with, and that people had noticed a new kind of illness in Wuhan.

Somehow, nearly the whole world misses the seemingly basic point of *this-is-an-idea*; the PCR test kits and our theories pertaining to their results are fallible, and the majority of civilians were reporting to each other heavily-hearted that "case numbers are soaring". No one ever said on the news that "positive cases are now *more likely* than they were last week ...", this would mean that whatever we are testing-for is growing in prevalence. To me, what would be appropriate to hear on the news at the start of such a thing as a 'pandemic' would be: "using the consistently randomised human-sampling and -testing method for detecting *microbe-X*, we have found positive cases are more prevalent than they were last week", and even then, bodily chemistry might just be moving along with the seasons and 'the microbe-X test' could've been passed with growing prevalence by the same humans the same time last year at the same rate... really we ought to be informed the pertinent details such as the increase in *disease itself* (and humidity/temperature/solar levels etc) comparative to the previous time last season, because the *X-diagnosis* itself may have only been made possible suddenly in the year the *X-pandemic* is apparent (as is/was the case with COVID19).

A messiah-machine—plague-watch, Bill Gates et al.'s best idea for using surplus resources—built upon a human delusion (contagion) has gone ahead and fired-up full-swing ... this is my best guess at this stage.

It seems to me that what has been documented as 'C19 virus' is actually just a newly documented measurement/analysis of human epithelial cell (lung cancer) particles/material: some human airway epithelial cells, in a Petrie dish, had a sample of material (said-virus-material inoculant) including antibiotics and centrifuged human respiratory liquid samples (3 humans' all who had pneumonia with no other theorised pneumonia-causing microbes detected in the usual PCR test): and the human epithelial cells broke down in a consequential fashion. The mock-inoculated cells received nothing, as far as I can tell: they didn't explicitly receive the antibiotics, and they definitely didn't receive any other kind of bio matter of a similar constitution to the alleged virus material (from the centrifuged samples). I don't think the antibiotics were used in the mock infection, because there was no contaminating bio-matter in the mock-infected cells, I'd say the mock cells underwent the same procedure only in being present within the same environment as the inoculated cells (minus the inoculant and antibiotics). I can't find verification on this from the address where I found the original study, not even in the supplementary index:

https://www.nejm.org/doi/full/10.1056/NEJMoa2001017 A Novel Coronavirus from Patients with Pneumonia in China, 2019 Na Zhu, Ph.D., Dingyu Zhang, M.D., Wenling Wang, Ph.D., Xingwang Li, M.D., Bo Yang, M.S., Jingdong Song, Ph.D., Xiang Zhao, Ph.D., Baoying Huang, Ph.D., Weifeng Shi, Ph.D., Roujian Lu, M.D., Peihua Niu, Ph.D., Faxian Zhan, Ph.D., et al., for the China Novel Coronavirus Investigating and Research Team

It could be that the antibiotics alone (regardless of the added biomatter that is likely to be an issue) is what causes the inoculated cells to form vesicles mistaken to be virus formations from infecting viruses. Maybe the inoculated cells received just 2x the amount of antibiotics, as I've seen before: Drs Mark and Sam Bailey have sported a great article, which includes discussion on exactly this point... they actually emailed the authors of the study which they assumed to be the main coronavirus isolation experiment (I was solely focussed on the other one from NEJM, and didn't know this one existed/took-place until later on thanks to the Bailey's), although it seems this one was published slightly after the one I was originally set-onto by Professor Vincent Racaniello (some days or weeks, regardless of the '20 February 2020' seemingly as part of the heading, it is written above the article on the NEJM website: "Editor's Note: This article was published on January 24, 2020, at NEJM.org." so I'm not sure who really had the more original one as the primary focus out of me and the Bailey's).

This is the study Drs M and S Bailey have thoroughly analysed: 'A pneumonia outbreak associated with a new coronavirus of probable bat origin' Peng Zhou, Xing-Lou Yang, Xian-Guang Wang, Ben Hu, Lei Zhang, Wei Zhang, Hao-Rui Si, Yan Zhu, Bei Li, Chao-Lin Huang, Hui-Dong Chen, Jing Chen, Yun Luo, Hua Guo, Ren-Di Jiang, Mei-Qin Liu, Ying Chen, Xu-Rui Shen, Xi Wang, Xiao-Shuang Zheng, Kai Zhao, Quan-Jiao Chen, Fei Deng, Lin-Lin Liu, Bing Yan, Fa-Xian Zhan, Yan-Yi Wang, Geng-Fu Xiao & Zheng-Li Shi published on the 3rd of February 2020 ... Dr Bailey's colleague reached-out to the author asking questions about what exactly was done to the control cells that were mock-inoculated... One co-author, Xing-Lou Yang, basically told them that the mock infected cells were treated with less antibiotics, as is evident and fully referenced in the following excerpt from Mark Bailey's 'A Farewell To Virology': https://drsambailey.com/a-farewell-to-virology-expert-edition/:

> "extracted some startling admissions from one of the paper's co-authors, Xing-Lou Yang. Firstly, aside from the fact that there were no positive control experiments (i.e. with comparable human samples minus the alleged virus), Yang stated they doubled the dose of penicillin and streptomycin in the experimental group. When asked why this variable was altered, the response was, "the intention 130 of Anti-Anti [the two antibiotics] is to prevent contamination from bacteria or fungi during virus isolation, so 1% or 2% concentration did not affect the cell growth. 2% in 1st gen [generation] was just to prevent contamination from samples."131 My colleague suggested that they should run the "control" experiment again with the higher dose antibiotics to ensure that this was not one of the factors inducing CPEs in the kidney cell line.

Yang subsequently provided the evasive response, "if you could make sure that you could prevent contamination from bac [bacteria] or fungi, you do not need to use the Anti-Anti," seemingly 132 ignoring the crucial point that it could be the additional antibiotics themselves that were toxic to the cells (particularly as streptomycin is known to be nephrotoxic). At the least, they had altered other variables compared with their controls and had thus invalidated their results even further.

Dr Mark Bailey's article clocks in at a whopping 67 pages of meticulously detailed analysis and investigation. Amongst other things (like PCR), he delves into the deep metagenomic sequencing (under the heading FAN WU ET AL. DEUS EX MACHINA), as it pertains to this big alleged delusion.

This next quote is from the NEJM coronavirus report, that I have spent hours focussed-on: "RNA extracted from bronchoalveolar-lavage fluid and culture supernatants was used as a template to clone and sequence the genome." Isolation of a virus in the usual sense does not result in one virus particle being analysed chemically or photographically, nor does the detection of it. And again, nor has any simulation of a natural encounter with any virus ever been shown to contribute to a cause of disease. Inoculating cellular cultures with bio-debris would likely be detrimental to the cells and cause them to break down faster than they would have had they not been *chemically contaminated*. Most pictures you see of so-called virus are CGI.

Most people assume a virus was isolated directly from human liquid samples, but this seemingly has never occurred: it seems *the Saliva Ocean* is too vast, therefore we seek to concentrate the cells the *alleged virus* infects—we make a lawn of the one kind of cell, add some materials to the lawn, and theorise ourselves to be propagating a virus that came from human liquid samples, otherwise we are just actioning the breakdown of cellular structures by *shattering their chemistry / malnourishing them* when we add our 'inoculant et al': we zoom in with a microscope and observe some destructive effect on the cells and harvest the remnants to be photographed. In this C19 case we see some rounded shapes that have resulted from the breakdown of once-viable cancer cells: from the resulting materials that muster during the breakdown of these cells, we run tests and photographs, and put together a model of genetic makeup and size and aesthetics for a theorised disease-causing virus (all from individual strands; not from one solid piece of genetic material is the virus modelled). I personally haven't learnt *precisely how* this resulting collection of material—alleged to be harvested C19 virus—has been biochemically analysed and put onto a map next to other materials alleged to be virus that have been biochemically analysed in the same way. I'm not sure how much of it is *made up*, but the molecular biologist Dr. Stefan Lanka probably is and he doesn't believe in self-replicating (let alone pathogenic) viruses. Perhaps the cells that break down in the experiment are from different sources with slightly differing genetics and they give-off a slightly different chemical reading, or they are processed differently before reading... maybe our lung epithelial cells are more chemically resemblant to bat lung epithelial cells than they are to some other kind of cell involved in our respiratory system, this would explain why some 'human coronaviruses' are alleged to be closer related to some 'bat coronaviruses' than other found 'human coronaviruses': remember all we can say as fact about viruses, is the type of cells and additives and process that has taken place to turn out the concoction/collection of material alleged to contain the theorised virus. I'm not compelled *to learn all the ways in which the big delusion has manifested*, I'm convinced I've naturally been compelled to learn more than enough and that the details I know just need to be laid-out in a certain way for thinkers to realise this really does seem beyond all reasonable doubt to be a major delusion, perhaps *the biggest*. The main take on why I don't believe in disease-causing viruses can be found in the Germ Theory part/chapter of this book.

Dr Lanka says he has made materials in his lab which pass as COVID19 under standard PCR detection, just with human cells containing no pathogens... it seems anyone who learns about this, assumes he has somehow found a flaw in the PCR method and is able *to trick it*, rather than concede something much bigger, like "*said COVID19 material* is wrought purely from human tissue, etc etc" ... his work is mostly in German but some is translated... I can only find an English-written report of the third phase... ... ... I don't really need it though, as well, to show any attentive normal person the overwhelming probability of *this big delusion*. The three phases of his experiment were — **Phase 1 – The cytopathic effect.** In the first control experiment, Dr. Stefan Lanka showed that what virologists attribute to the presence of a pathogenic virus can be achieved without infectious material. A report to phase 1 can be found in German (https://coldwelliantimes.com/eilmeldung/kontrollexperiment-phase-1-mehrere-labore-bestatigen-die-widerlegung-der-virologie-durch-den-cytopathischen-effekt/). — **Phase 2 – Construction of the SARS-CoV-2 genome.** In the second control experiment, Dr. Lanka showed that what virologists call "viral genetic material actually comes from a healthy human tissue. - https://www.youtube.com/watch?v=gtWri6FvG14 — **Phase 3 – Structural analysis of sequency data in virology.** In the third control experiment, we show that with the same technique that virologists use and using nucleic acids, which are not from supposedly infectious material but from healthy human tissue, animals and plants, can construct the genome of any "virus." - *an actual report in English* **is published here** for this finding: https://viroliegyhome.files.wordpress.com/2022/08/structural_analysis_of_sequence_data_in_virology28129.pdf I suspect Dr Lanka of not wanting all the full reports out there for any of us to use in our books etc, at this stage, whilst there has been no significant change in worldwide belief re contagious diseases, otherwise he'd hurriedly pump out English version of the

116

reports from phase 1 and 2 too, and like I said phase 1 can be found in German (https://coldwelliantimes.com/eilmeldung/kontrollexperiment-phase-1-mehrere-labore-bestatigen-die-widerlegung-der-virologie-durch-den-cytopathischen-effekt/) and phase 2 report seemingly doesn't exist at all yet he's come out and told us of the outcomes... he probably thinks there's no way any of us can settle the debate if he can't, and he actually wants to be the one who settles it (lord knows he has done a lot of work labouring under the stress of condemnation by his peers in academia). Maybe Dr Lanka is keeping phase 2 report for his team solely to use in a legal matter, before letting it out to the rest of the world (maybe he thinks the legal matter will lead to the major belief for humanity).

I don't think Stefan Lanka or any of the other prominent thinkers in this situation, like Dr T Cowan, have enough natural respect for it, and I find them frustrating to listen-to when I imagine myself as a sincere-believer in germ/virus theory (Richard Dawkins, who is perhaps my personal single-most educational benefactor via his books) who happens to stumble upon their talks about it, and this is essentially why I think they haven't yet changed the world … they are speaking with an average level of specific empathy and a lot of excitement and *seemingly offence*, they have not the emotional intelligence to discuss these things in a way that is bridging for people who haven't happened to view an array of info that has appealed to them and allowed for the intellectual opening/whetting for further induction… and, as I said, I think Lanka is holding back from sharing with us immediately everything so as to minimise the chances of someone else becoming prominent for effecting a major dominoes-like change in belief (I've personally been ignored)—imagining he is most-fit to effect all the influence that would come with such a prominence.

All the pertinent data I have checked is well and truly congruent with the idea of there being nothing new in terms of human potential to pass as positive within the same PCR detection process being used all over the world for the C19 operation, and I bet there is not one study online available where people have sought to test whether any bio samples existing before August 2019 can pass as positive for COVID19, because we don't have enough people thinking in that direction to call for such a study. The fluctuating testing efforts and protocols in the areas that have 'outbreaks of cases', is seemingly the primary cause of the increase in case numbers in those areas: teams hypothesise an outbreak at spot-X, and then go and run increased tests at spot-X then say "look, our hypothesis ... we were right ... ". The humans cash-in on morale when they believe their supervisors saw an outbreak coming and made it so much better than it otherwise would've been ... no one has ever mentioned that an outbreak occurred whilst there was a consistent testing effort in place well before and during the outbreak. This whole C19 operation is a great exposé.

During the developing days of the C19 world operation, it seems to be accepted in the background that if you are capable of producing a specimen that will pass positive, you will be recognised and thusly tested, hence many people thought they could calculate a case-fatality ratio for the alleged microbe.

https://www.nejm.org/doi/full/10.1056/NEJMoa2001017

Here is an excerpt from the original NEJM study, which I've found quite telling:

> In late December 2019, several local health facilities reported clusters of patients with pneumonia of unknown cause that were epidemiologically linked to a seafood and wet animal wholesale market in Wuhan, Hubei Province, China.11 On December 31, 2019, the Chinese Center for Disease Control and Prevention (China CDC) dispatched a rapid response

team to accompany Hubei provincial and Wuhan city health authorities and to conduct an epidemiologic and etiologic investigation.

This is admitting that the rationale to *investigate and sequence the theorised genome of some specimens* was anecdotal—that is to say, there was no *reported data* of a sudden increase in respiratory illness, and no reported data of an increase in the ratio/amount of unknown viral pneumonia cases that were being diagnosed (if there was, this is precisely the paragraph that should/would tell us).

If you think the fact that coronaviruses were being studied in a lab in Wuhan is strong evidence that it was Chinese people who developed and released the hypothetical bio-weapon, I invite you to consider the opposite just as well (that the Chinese people would be the last to blame, assuming they wouldn't want to be blamed for it).

In spite of all this, Italy and Bulgaria and more countries in Europe began to experience an extraordinarily high mortality rate for their older population, which coincided with the beginning of the lockdowns in these countries, to name a few. Bulgaria and Italy were having arguably the greatest recorded year ever in mortality until the weeks the lockdowns started, and as the lockdown started it appears as though the Bulgarian and Italian children began to experience record-low mortality rates and the elderly experience record-high. If you're wondering where I got these data leads from, it's all at https://www.mortality.org/. I've seen refined data from this website. The article in this link references more precisely and broadly what I have just discussed in this paragraph: https://vaccinationdilemma.com/2021/05/20/covid-19-part-6-comparing-2020-death-rates-with-previous-years-continued/#comment-11749.

Where's the new antibody?

We should be testing blood samples from pre-August 2019 and talking about that. No one seems to be catering for this point: Where is the distinct line for the new kinds of antibodies that started developing? Can we find it in the blood bank? Some people have had a little look: Unexpected detection of SARS-CoV-2 antibodies in the pre-pandemic period in Italy https://doi.org/10.1177/0300891620974755 ...

No line of distinction has been observed at this stage. Although September 2019 is not that long ago, this *seems to be* the earliest blood samples anyone has taken the time to test for C19 antibodies, and the antibodies are there, yet C19 wasn't even officially recognised at this stage. The three samples the C19 signature was established from were analysed in December 2019.

What should have occurred once the C19 signature was established in Wuhan was a rapid response to collect a heap of other patients' samples from around the world with pneumonia of unknown cause (and even known, as I'm sure you can have more than one kind of disease-associated particle in you), to observe if any of them harboured the C19 signature. Instead, we waited several weeks or months, shrieking "Is it here yet?" before the world developed readily accessible test kits and started off on an exponentially-growing testing campaign, shrieking "Case numbers are now soaring!". The world is not owned and orchestrated by a scientist, but currently it is moved around by many ideas alleging to be scientific; The Gates foundation appears here more focussed on 'saving humanity' than science (perhaps that would make a famous billionaire in a world full of poverty feel good enough about his *raison d'etre*).

Apparently, most of the indigenous people in Australia and America died after European invasion, and apparently the primary reason was "they encountered a microbe they hadn't yet encountered". COVID19 was said to be causing pneumonia, and no human had encountered it until 2019 in Wuhan when it evolved inside a bat (or in a lab, or wherever) to the point where it was able to infect humans. Both Korea and Taiwan experienced record low mortality rates for the year 2020, according to https://www.mortality.org/.

As for vaccination:

I've reviewed the Moderna (https://youtu.be/doTkPRxMAFA and https://www.youtube.com/watch?v=Jg91dNRM4Nc), Astra Zeneca, and Pfizer vaccine trial reports (https://youtu.be/eiTxuCfzHoY), and there's nothing new here, as they specifically *still* haven't lowered a measure of overall disease-incidence or mortality when comparing to no placebo injection or else simple saline-solution placebo injection. The Astra Zeneca vaccine was reported to have lowered hospital admissions, which is to say nothing for vaccination itself because all the humans in the control/placebo group were vaccinated with a meningococcal vaccine instead of the COVID vaccine in order that they may not know if they received the COVID vaccine under trial, *as a placebo control* (https://www.thelancet.com/journals/lancet/article/PIIS0140-6736(20)32661-1/fulltext).

Why were people circa 2021 saying that these vaccines haven't been tested well enough yet? The question, to me, is nonsensical, because it implies that an uncontrolled period of observation is a legitimate form of a test or experiment for such a product, and it implies that other vaccines on the infant schedule have been more thoroughly tested for safety and efficacy. These vaccines have been tested just as thoroughly as ones available at your local clinic before COVID19. The MRNA technology may be the reason people are saying this, but there are other things to worry about which we haven't as thoroughly tested from other vaccines added to the infant schedule and even air pollutants and water additives that have probably been tested less thoroughly than these MRNA vaccines—these were not the first nanoparticle-employing vaccines. The longest time a vaccine has been observed for safety and effectiveness under controlled observations, that I have found, is 2.5 years. That was in Japan, 2009–2012. I've covered it in this book, and I don't recall anyone talking about it on the news as if we as a culture had thus learnt something more about vaccination per se.

Epilogue

On the ambiguity of antibodies

As I briefly discussed in 'The Flu Vaccine' chapter: as far as I can tell, there is no clarification that there are specific tailor-made antibodies... perhaps some team managed to test these primer ingredients (used for detecting specific antibodies in blood samples) to be sure that they highlight specifically-exclusive features of immunoglobulin specific only to a particular antibody which was made only for a particular antigen which pertains to a particular character of disease: if this study or clarification has been achieved, I am not sure why I can't find it or no one like the PhD virologist and molecular biologist Dr S Lanka talks about it, he seems to simply claim that it's nearly all imaginary modelling. It is my contention that these primers used at this stage, are not well-controlled, they are haphazard ingredients included and are unique in themselves when compared to each of the different ingredients/primers used in each different antibody test, and this helps effect the illusion that they help us detect special antibodies which the body makes specifically for a particular antigen that can rapidly multiply itself in the body, amongst a plethora of other kinds of antibodies/antigens (key/lock).

No antibody has ever been isolated itself. It seems all we have proof-of, regarding antibodies, is that immunoglobulin production is spiked during cellular reparation and obstruction, especially when highly-adjuvanted vaccines are given. We seem to—in all of these vaccine-trials where recipients are screened for the given antibody as a marker of vaccine effectiveness, and any time someone is tested for a specific antibody—have no clarification that we aren't only measuring a spike of immunoglobulin: it seems we can't be sure that antibodies as we imagine them even exist... although, the assessment of vaccination effectiveness and contagious disease is unscathed by this nebula: whether there are truly-matched antigen-antibody couples whereby the tailor-made antibody even waits around to be coupled-up *only with the given antigen*, or whether we have a of range of immunoglobulin that we employ to grab/clean the things that cause chemical imbalance and obstruction to our physiology and patch up areas that need bonding/mending, does not matter when assessing precisely what has vaccination demonstrated and precisely what has been pronounced in terms of disease-causation. I have carried out my assessment of vaccination and contagion, with the benefit of the doubt granted that there really are key/lock specific-antibody formations, although I currently am not a believer. Here is a link to the most detailed account I have found on the history and genesis of antibody-theory, which I have already shared in an earlier chapter: https://viroliegy.com/category/antibodies/ Note how this website has a play on the word 'lie'? I don't particularly like the emphasis on lie, because this gives a false impression that the whole thing is essentially a lie rather than delusion. I believe lies are told by people generally in the form of false-assurance rather than conscious contradiction of information: the alternative to the big delusion here would be the big lie, which would involve people deliberately inseminating an maintaining the idea of vaccination and germ theory when they truly themselves believe against these ideas. People lie about things they truly believe in, like the chemist who assured me "the WHO" has ran a well-controlled trial that showed vaccinated humans endured significantly less adversity or mortality than unvaccinated humans.

Death

It seems every cell itself has an end stage that is reached one way or another (regardless of allegedly-immortal cell lines, the individual cells themselves wither away). Not every organism reproduces, and the determining factors of whether an organism will reproduce (the things which make it easy/hard) are constantly changing fast or slow. There is always this scene of competition and cooperation between organisms. Whether the organisms are consciously competing or not, and whether or not they are making a strenuous effort, probably does not truly correlate with reproductive success: successful reproduction proceeds most often not through every sexually mature organism in the field, but through those that are fitting within the present circumstances (the ones who try the hardest may be the least successful, in general). The environment, the ecosystem, the weather, the neighbours— these circumstances are constantly changing, fast or slow. Nothing is fixated in the natural world. Along with the changing circumstances goes changing ideas, changing value of ideas, and the changing value for different kinds of organisms who take up these ideas and carry them out in their own unique way. Two major circumstance changers in human history: the mastery of fire, and contraception.

I personally ultimately identify as existence, so technically it seems I do not actually die. I do not ultimately identify as thought or memory or any particular tissue/material at any particular time or location.

War

A group of humans that were subdued 10 thousand years ago may have been more fitting in today's circumstances to conquer the world—are they an inferior race of humans just because they lost a war in those circumstances 10k years ago? Is a group superior in some outright sense if it can beat another group right now? What if the more depressed less-happy group of humans more often plans and wins wars? Superiority, value, potential—these are circumstantially relative concepts regarding an organism. If a person doesn't feel good, or do much, or have many resources, or have any friends or sexual partners, in the dawn of the 21st century, does this mean that organism is inferior-to and not-as-fit as a human who has loads of money and sexual partners and friends and is full of vigour at the same time and place? These things are circumstantial, and the human who had no friends or sexual partners might even be having the superior experience in consciousness... and thus winners of wars could be of a lower existential value only appearing as a readjustment feature of human settlements/cultures/activity... I think we should nowadays start something unprecedented.

Life

As the current paradigm of humanity is unsustainable, the circumstances need to change. Although they will and are changing, serious thinkers on the subject of global sustainability suggest this needs to happen much faster. The new circumstances of life that will emerge will be suitable and more fitting to a different kind of human that currently doesn't find itself thriving in these tumultuous conditions. There is no outright/objective superiority or inferiority in form itself.

Humanity should be more enchanted by the fact of 10000 years from now. We should be gracefully sending-it with that kind of fact in mind, and enjoying good-feelings of how we are creating the future kind-of how we feel good/engaged/*moved* watching a soap opera, we can visualise the future occurring: "it is a fact that *something* will be happening in 10000 years (no such thing as nothing) ... it is a fact that whatever will be happening is a result of what's happening right now = What are we doing? Do we have any pressing concerns?" = Build asteroid-destroying/-diverting technology, establish and secure a stable and healthy path of existence (hobbies and all) within the earth's ecosystem for humanity. All of this would involve the coordination of the entire human collective, which doesn't mean we all have to be living the same lifestyle under the same rules—we can have district and global votes on what is and isn't allowed to happen (majority-voting leads) within districts and globally—we need to be *the same force of power*. Debating, thinking, influencing will be the new martial frontier, the new front line = "we must change these people's minds before the vote!".

Currently, with the global human network, with extended nation-families (countries), with the elaborate systems of labour and social welfare, it has become really easy for the average human to reproduce without having to perform to the best of its ability, without having to really dig into the potential of its efforts. In times of plenty, a lineage should be building up its *power*, and it seems we have no responsibility for ourselves because in this time of plenty most people are opting to fill their stomachs on MacDonald's burgers and drink sugary carbonated and caffeinated water (food-drugs), partying... Mohammad (the prophet of Islam (peace be upon him)) was noted for saying that man abuses his stomach more than any other organ, and he lived well before the fast-food revolution. Things have become colossal regarding humans abusing their stomachs ...

Since the agricultural revolution, the mass provision of vitamin-D-deficient nutriment (grains) became widely practised (and put a selection-pressure on humans with lighter skin who can make their own vitamin-D more efficiently than the darker-skinned humans; grain-eating culture seems to be the key selection pressure for those with lighter skin, really only in areas with not *too much* sun), and many human populations based on this mono-cropping grain-storing culture grew to large numbers very quickly (heaps of human births and deaths ... lots of disease occurred for these rapidly-erecting grain-based civilisations). Grain can store for a long time and has a high yield-rate per hectare for dried foods. This was the birth of the common class, the majority of people: fed by the system which is implemented, supervised and maintained by a respected political class/monarchy, with everybody having the same reproductive capability (more or less), so long as you participated in society. The common people were encouraged to reproduce under the specified rules of their society, none of which selected-for a *more* accurately-calculating or physically-superior organism than the previous lifestyle/culture, rather selecting-for features like obedience and socio-emotional-callousness.

The rapid expansion of the human gene pool, particularly after the agricultural revolution, expanded from a group of humans that was only there to expand-upon because they and their ancestors had a certain make-up which allowed for successful reproduction in their pre-agriculture circumstances: the *average* member of this pre-grain group may very well have been more precisely calculating (perspicacious and sagacious) and physically superior, representing value to the group in collecting, supervising navigating and defending, and also in leading group-cohesion/inspiration stories.

Power

It is not a new thing that a population of organisms may experience such an incredible suspense in survival and reproductive pressure—it happened for the second time to a walking, talking fire-harbouring mammal who thenceforth grew even more floppy-eared so to speak, and maybe not as superior physically and mentally (on average). It has currently been estimated that this occurred circa 10,000 BC (true farming).

From the point of being able to feed thousands under the one umbrella with farming technology, the human gene pool grew from the foundational humans who brought about the technology and system, bursting into many civilisations based on grain farming. The way that it grew was not free from any impediments: it wasn't as if every kind of human found the life of deep-subordination (*to people you aren't familiar with*), obedience, grain-eating, monotonous labour and the particular rules of the society fitting for their reason for existence. Without this reason for existence satisfied—without the zest for life—the human won't be so apt to go out to work daily, to rear a family and participate in society, or to go to war. Such a selection pressure, some have argued, is a selection for a duller, less-brainy, obedient labourer who is happy to live and work amongst many humans who are unfamiliar yet are in the same group. The domesticated homo sapiens: faithful and obedient beasts. It is my opinion that a naturally-selected form of retardation has set-in upon homo sapiens since this agricultural-civilisation trajectory formed: a form of emotional and intellectual retardation that laid out the path for an exponential expansion of the collective human body/power: the cultural machine of the collective societies did grow more sophisticated and powerful, and has afforded us humans higher luxuries/life and the ability to sport super-knowledgeable members with unprecedented powers. These agricultural cultures superseded the other cultures in sheer numbers on the battlefield. Again, the primary motivation was not simply to destroy, but to maintain, to allow for breeding (a sense of survival) to continue, to preserve by eliminating possible threats and resource-leaks.

Our major priority for the human race should be to accept the responsibility of owning the earth and cleaning it up and keeping it clean. Currently, from the air to the ocean, *this place is a mess*, and we need to quit warring and start repairing. We are wise enough now from all our lessons, and we have the technology—we shall capitulate.

We need to accept imperfection: Already, there is the chance for injustice to be playing out at all our elections and basically anywhere official. We need to pre-arrange the conditions with all of this in mind, all the facts of the situation, accepting imperfection, and capitulate. The only rational system of politics is a majority-vote system, all the rest are tyrannical in nature because they require some humans to have absolutely no say for no reason, and no human or small group of them is infallible; we all should take responsibility for ourselves and our neighbours, from how many kids an adult can have in a given district to how many kids districts can allow people to have under what circumstances. Trust the voting machine, the messiah—what's the alternative? The messiah will obviously be an AI that mediates for humanity and gives us insight into what the majority votes are, for what and where, and for what we need to be thinking/voting about next.

Order

You simply cannot say that some other human adult is dumber than you and you will vote for them: to me, this is the major lesson Jesus gives us. You cannot rule over the consciousness of another human being, which is what occurs when some humans decide officially that other humans are inferior in judgement. Elitism needs to stop as we have no proof that this ever isn't actually a form of parasitism. You cannot say that you are better than someone, and that they can't vote, unless the person has been officially recognised and accepted within the community in accordance to prearranged (voted-in/on) guidelines. If humanity is so dumb it needs an elite to rule it, then we can't be confident that that's actually what's happening (that they are actually 'elite' rather than high-strung con artists): humanity can lead itself, smart people can try to teach dumb people, and we can be dignified to know we all together steer this ship not just a small group of people who manage to tell us all that they naturally are our ruling elite and our best chance at societal and cultural navigation. No one person should have more say than anyone else, ideas should have more votes: if people are so smart and/or wise, and/or powerful, they can still change the culture/minds and perhaps in a much more insight-stimulating manner for the culture... this could be a very good thing that makes the average person more able to think about things, this could make it more popular to discuss and think about ideas.

If I know nothing about *fracking*, and I'm called upon to vote on whether or not we can do it, I will take whatever information I am inclined to gather and vote yes or no accordingly, whether I make my decision based on the look of someone's face when they tell me they know something about it, whether I simply like one billboard better than another, or if I base a vote on a highly elaborate personal calculation of pollutive materials and future sustainability and current requirements and values ...

One way to avoid corruption would be to lose secrecy in voting and show for your vote in a way that means you can be held accountable for it by anyone involved in the voting—and why should we keep this secret? We should all be able to form up online with our votes, and take responsibility to screen anyone present for illegitimacy, and know that we-all-know who is who through all the interconnected groups that can keep themselves and each other off, through the extended social network, we can pull-card anywhere we need to... if someone doesn't want to let people know which way they are voting, then maybe that's a good reason to not let them vote on a communal decision. This is our culture and we need to look after it and each other, there's no reason we should facilitate sneak-voting, we all can be better than that: if it's a public issue it's a public issue. Or we can accept imperfection and trust the AI or human contractors counting the votes, and keep secrecy. I think we ought to become one "world power" rather than many nations, and focus our resources and energy on policing ourselves better rather than preparing to fight. I bet this would create and sustain a more diverse, progressive and exciting life for humanity, we would have much more resources available... we waste so much energy and opportunity because apparently we can't all get along with each other, and I mean: nearly no person seems to intuit just how much resources and energy is wasted and not-accumulated because we simply are in this multi-national competition... I also am convinced that more security can lead to more privacy, and better policing affords higher freedom, and we are accepting a very low standard of these essential communal functions due to our us-and-them struggle on this ancient battlefield: we can't afford that high of a standard for ourselves, because of the big scary battlefield dynamics we sport a military, this is probably 70% of our energy: military muscle constantly being exercised and flexed destroying ecosystems). We should only have WOMD for handling incoming asteroids/comets.

Humans should be thriving in a truly democratic society, with global voting on world-rules (what regions can and can't

131

police/do), and regional voting (what the specific region wants to police/do). We shouldn't be stressing about wasted opportunities and resources and failing ecosystems. A world that is fragmented in power is irresponsible for itself as a whole, and the fragmented powers will compete with each other and cut moral corners to survive in the obvious short-term ...

I rest my case.

This book is available for purchase on Amazon, you can find it through googling the title and author. You can contact me at lewis.beattie92@gmail.com or at the Facebook page named Vaccination Elucidation. I also have a YouTube channel named Powersend (https://www.youtube.com/@powersend).

Printed in Great Britain
by Amazon

16627660R00078